CW00739802

A Straight

Being a Mental Health
Service User

A Straight Talking Introduction to

Being a Mental Health Service User

Peter Beresford

PCCS BOOKS
Ross-on-Wye

First published 2010

PCCS BOOKS Ltd
2 Cropper Row
Alton Road
Ross-on-Wye
Herefordshire
HR9 5LA
UK
Tel +44 (0)1989 763900
www.pccs-books.co.uk

**A Straight Talking Introduction to
Being a Mental Health Service User**

A CIP catalogue record for this book is available from the British Library

ISBN 978 1 906254 20 9

Cover designed in the UK by Old Dog Graphics
Typeset in the UK by The Old Dog's Missus
Printed in the UK by Ashford Colour Press, Gosport, Hampshire

Contents

Dedication

This book is dedicated to all the mental health service users/survivors I have met, on my own journey through the system and through service user organisations, who are no longer with us. People like me owe them a lot. It is also dedicated to those still making or who have yet to make that journey, wishing them my best and every support possible.

Acknowledgements

There are many people to thank for their help in writing this book. First the group of mental health service users/ survivors from whom I have quoted who came together to help inform the book through their discussion: Lucia Franco, Adrian Tibbs, Colin Dean and John Clark. Then the survivors who I have quoted individually in the book who were all kind enough to put down their views for me to include. I'd also like to thank Wendy Bryant from Brunel University, Pete Sanders from PCCS Books, for his patience and encouragement (that may not be strong enough a word!) and Sandy Green from PCCS Books for her sensitive editing which has improved the book. Also Louise Pembroke and Peter Campbell for the longstanding understanding and inspiration I have gained from them, as well as the Survivors' History Group and electronic website for the constant insights I have gained from them. My thanks also to Simon Kewer for his illustrations for the book and Jan Wallcraft for her foreword. Most of all of course I would like to thank the many people who have given me support and helped me to gain understanding through my experience of madness and distress and the mental health system and all those people who have helped make the survivor movement what it is. Thank you.

Introduction to the *Straight Talking* series

What are mental health problems?

Much of what is written and spoken about emotional distress or mental health problems implies that they are illnesses. This can lead us all too easily to believe that we no longer have to think about mental health problems, because illness is best left to doctors. They are the illness experts, and psychiatrists are the doctors who specialise in mental illness. This series of books is different because we don't think that all mental health problems should be automatically regarded as illnesses.

If mental health problems aren't necessarily illnesses, it means that the burden of responsibility for distress in our lives should not be entirely shouldered by doctors and psychiatrists. All citizens have a responsibility, however small, in creating a world where everyone has a decent opportunity to live a fulfilling life. This is a contentious idea, but one which we want to advance alongside the dominant medical view.

Rather than accept that solutions to mental health problems are 'owned' by the medical profession, we will take a good look at alternatives which involve the users of psychiatric services, their carers, families, friends and other 'ordinary people' taking control of their own lives. One of the tools required in order to become active in mental health issues, whether your own or other people's, is knowledge. This series of books is a starting point for anyone who wants to know more about mental health.

How these books are written

We want these books to be understandable, so we use everyday language wherever possible. The books could have been almost completely jargon-free, but we thought that including some technical and medical terms would be helpful. Most doctors, psychiatrists and psychologists use the medical model of mental illness and manuals to help them diagnose mental health problems. The medical model and the diagnostic manuals use a particular set of terms to describe what doctors think of as 'conditions'. Although these words aren't very good at describing individual people's experiences, they are used a lot in psychiatric and psychological services, so we thought it would be helpful to define these terms as we went along and use them in a way that might help readers understand what the professionals mean. We don't expect that psychiatrists and psychologists and others working in mental health services will stop using medical terminology (although we think it might be respectful for them to drop it when talking to their patients and their families), so these books should help you get used to, and learn *their* language.

At the end of the book on p. 137 there are some contacts and resources. There are also endnotes and although these will not be important to everyone they do tell the reader where information – a claim about effectiveness, an argument for or against, or a quotation – has come from so you can follow it up if you wish.

Being realistic and reassuring

Our aim is to be realistic – neither overly optimistic nor pessimistic. Things are nearly always more complicated than we would like them to be. Honest evaluations of mental health problems, of what might cause them, of what can help, and of what the likely outcome might be, are, like so much in life, somewhere in between. For the vast majority of people it would be wrong to say that they have an illness from which they will never recover. But it would be equally wrong to say that they will be completely unchanged by the distressing thoughts and feelings they are having. Life is an accumulation of experiences. There is usually no pill, or any other treatment for that matter, that will take us back to 'how we were before'. There are many things we can do (and we will be looking at lots of them in this series) in collaboration with doctors, psychiatrists, psychologists, counsellors, indeed everyone working in mental health services, with the help of our friends and family, or on our own, which stand a good chance of helping us feel better and build a constructive life with hope for the future.

Of course, we understand that the experiences dealt with in these books can sometimes be so overwhelming, confusing and terrifying that people will try to escape from them by withdrawing, going mad or even by trying to kill themselves. This happens when our usual coping strategies fail us. We accept that killing oneself is, in some circumstances, a rational act – that for the person in question it can make a lot of sense. Nonetheless, we believe that much of the distress that underpins such an extreme course of action, from which there can be no turning back, is avoidable. For this reason, all of the books in this series point towards realistic hope and recovery.

Debates

There is no single convenient answer to many of the most important questions explored in these books. No matter how badly we might wish for a simple answer, what we have is a series of debates, or arguments more like, between stakeholders and there are many stakeholders whose voices demand space in these books. We use the word 'stakeholders' here because service users, carers, friends, family, doctors, psychologists, psychiatrists, nurses and other workers, scientists in drug companies, therapists, indeed all citizens, have a stake in how our society understands and deals with problems of mental health. It is simultaneously big business and intimately personal, and many things in between. As we go along, we try to explain how someone's stake in distress (including our own, where we can see it), whether business or personal, can influence their experience and judgement.

Whilst we want to present competing (sometimes opposing) viewpoints, we don't want to leave the reader high and dry to evaluate complicated debates on their own. We will try to present reasonable conclusions which might point in certain directions for personal action. Above all, though, we believe that knowledge is power and that the better informed you are, even though the information might be conflicting, the more able you will be to make sound decisions.

It's also useful to be reminded that the professionals involved in helping distressed people are themselves caught in the same flow of conflicting information. It is their *job*, however, to interpret it in our service, so that the best solutions are available to as many people as possible. You may have noticed that the word 'best' brings with it certain challenges, not least of all, what we mean when we use this term. Perhaps the best means the most effective? However, even using words like 'effective' doesn't completely clear up the puzzle. An effective treatment could be the one which returns someone to work quickly, if you are an employer, or one which makes someone feel happier and more calm, if they are your son or daughter. Readers will also know from recent press coverage that the National Institute for Health and Clinical Excellence (NICE), which evaluates and recommends treatments, keeps one eye on the budget, so 'effective' might mean 'cost effective' to some people. This brings us to evidence.

Evidence

Throughout these books there will be material which we will present as 'evidence'. This is one of the most contentious terms to be found in this series. One person's evidence is another person's fanciful mythology and yet another person's oppressive propaganda. Nevertheless the term crops up increasingly in everyday settings, most relevantly when we hear of 'evidence-based practice'. The idea behind this term is that the treatments psychologists and psychiatrists offer should be those that work. Crudely put, there should be some evidence that, say, talking about problems, or taking a prescribed drug, actually helps people to feel better. We encounter a real problem however, when trying to evaluate this evidence, as the books will demonstrate. We will try not to discount any 'evidence' out of hand, but we will evaluate it, and we will do this with a bias towards scientific evaluation.

The types of evidence that will be covered in these books, along with their positive and negative points, include the following.

Research methods, numbers and statistics

On the one hand, the logic of most research is simple, but on the other hand, the way things have to be arranged to avoid bias in the results can lead to a perplexing system of measurements. Even the experts lose the sense of it sometimes. We'll try to explain the logic of studies, but almost certainly leave out the details. You can look these up yourself if you wish.

The books in this series look at research into a wide range of issues regarding mental health problems, including the experience of distress, what is known about the causes of problems, and their prevention and treatment. Different research methods are more or less appropriate for each of these areas, so we will be looking at different types of research as we go along. We say this now because many readers may be most familiar with studies into the *effective treatments* of distress, and we want to emphasise that there are many credible and valid sources of essential information about distress that are sometimes overlooked.

You may have come across the idea that some research methods are 'better' than others – that they constitute a 'gold standard'. In the case of research into the effectiveness of different treatments, the gold standard is usually considered to be 'randomised controlled trials' (RCTs). In simple terms, RCTs are complex (and often very expensive) experiments in which a group of individuals who all suffer from the same problem are randomly allocated to a treatment or a 'control' condition (at its simplest, no treatment at all) to see whether the treatment works. We are not necessarily convinced that RCTs always *are* the best way of conducting research into effective treatments, but they are, at the present time, the method given most credence by bodies which control funding, such as the National Health Service's National Institute of Health and Clinical Excellence (NICE), so we need to understand them.

Personal experience

Personal experience is an important source of evidence to the extent that nowadays, people who have suffered debilitating psychiatric distress are sometimes called 'experts by experience'.

Personal stories provide an essential counterbalance to the impersonal numbers and statistics often found in research projects such as RCTs. Whilst not everyone is average, by definition, most people are. Balancing the average results obtained from RCTs with some personal stories helps complete the picture and is now widely accepted to the extent that it has given birth to the new field of 'survivor research'.

Understanding contexts

Widening our view to include the families and lives of people, and the cultural, economic, social and political settings in which we live completes the picture. Mental health problems are connected to the conditions in which we all live, just as much as they are connected to our biology. From the start we want readers to know that, if there is one message or model which the books are trying to get across, it is that problems in mental health are more often than not the result of complex events in the environments in which we live and our reactions to them. These reactions can also be influenced by our biology or the way we have learned to think and feel. Hopefully these books will help disentangle the puzzle of distress and provide positive suggestions and hope for us all, whether we work in the system, currently have mental health problems ourselves, are caring for someone or are friends with someone who has.

We hope that readers of these books will feel empowered by what they learn, and thereby more able to get the best out of mental health services. It would be wonderful if our efforts, directly or indirectly, influence the development of services that effectively address the emotional, social and practical needs of people with mental health problems.

Richard Bentall
Pete Sanders
April 2009

Foreword
Jan Wallcraft

Peter Beresford has been an inspiration to me and to many other service users/survivors as we try to make sense of our lives in this 'maddening' world.[1]

All Peter's work and writing is done openly as someone who has experienced mental distress and psychiatric treatment. He works consistently to challenge medical assumptions about mental distress and psychiatric labelling, and to help people to take power over their own lives.

Peter is never afraid to be controversial, but does not make cheap points to get headlines. He always ensures that his work is based on the lived experience of mental health service users and disabled people. He writes in language which is free from jargon and clearly sets out the views of a wide range of people who have been on the receiving end of state services.

Many of us have reason to be thankful for the articles he has written in the Guardian, his dedicated work to involve service users and carers in social work policy and education, and his commitment to supporting service user-led research.

Straight talking is indeed needed, so is the openness and courage which Peter himself models in his work.

This book is timely, coming at a point in history when a new government is intent on changing the landscape of mental health and social services yet again, with renewed attacks on so-called 'benefits scroungers' and those with long-term needs for services and support.

This book is based on Peter's interviews with service users, and a wide range of research evidence.

As is pointed out throughout this book, it is not rare to have mental health problems, or to be a friend or family member of someone who does; yet mental health problems are still widely misunderstood, resulting in those who have a problem with their mental health being afraid to ask for help. Many of those who receive treatment do not find it helpful, and many end up feeling excluded because of the attitudes of others.

The book guides the reader through the 'parallel universe' of the mental health system, and explains the mental health service user/survivor movement set up to challenge our exclusion from the mainstream. It explores issues for a range of minority groups who often face even worse discrimination and exclusion.

It looks at how service users share support and information, advocate for one another, get involved in trying to change the system and create alternatives. It explores how social models of disability and mental health are posing a fundamental challenge to exclusion, by developing concepts such as independent living with ongoing support as needed.

Finally, Peter sets out a vision for the future, acknowledging that it is not just the psychiatric system, but the world that needs changing. He sets out key principles for change, which can be achieved if we work together, as individuals taking back our own power, and through our networks and alliances.

This book offers valuable information, a message of hope and a call for collective action for real, sustainable change through practical strategies such as rights-based, anti-oppressive practice, support for independent living, building the capacity of service user groups, and enabling service user-led research and services. I wish it had been available when I was beginning my own recovery from mental distress and psychiatric treatment, and I hope it is widely read and shared by mental health service users and survivors and those who care for or about them.

Dr Jan Wallcraft
Survivor researcher; Honorary Fellow, University of Birmingham;
Visiting Fellow, University of Hertfordshire

Introduction to this book

> I believe in the need to generate knowledge from the
> perspective of the least powerful groups in society. Within
> mental health research, this means discovery and
> exploration with and for the people who use and refuse
> psychiatric services.[1]
> *Angela Sweeney*

The aim of this book is to talk clearly and openly about an
issue that is highly contentious and which raises strong
emotions, particularly fear. There is no agreed terminology
in this field, instead there is talk of mental health problems,
madness, mental illness and distress, as well as the routine
use of many demeaning terms like 'nutter' and 'loony'. This
is a book about making sense of being a mental health
service user. It is an issue in which many people and groups
have an interest: policymakers, politicians, economists,
professionals, family, friends and loved ones and, of course,
service users themselves. Thus interest may arise for
occupational, political, financial, academic or personal
reasons. The reasons people directly experiencing madness
and distress have for such interest – people now increasingly
called 'service users' or survivors – are the most direct and
can be expected to be the most intense. Historically,
however, they have also been the most devalued and least
documented. Yet mental health service users/survivors have
unique experience, knowledge and understanding to offer.

That is why this book not only focuses on being a mental health service user, but is also written by and from the perspective of a mental health service user.

Interest in the perspectives of mental health service users/survivors reflects a broader policy and political interest in the views and experience of people on the receiving end of policy and politics. In recent years in the UK and internationally, there has been a new interest in 'user-centred' and 'user-led' practice and provision in many areas of policy, from education and health, to housing and leisure. There has been an official interest in involving service users, consulting with them and listening to their views. We will look more at the reasons for this later. But this raises some particular issues in relation to mental health services and mental health service users which need to be considered carefully. This is because mental health policy can and does restrict people's rights, as well as providing support. Mental health service users are still frequently seen as threatening and dangerous, as well as people who need help. This raises questions about how we can make involvement and user-led services real for this group and how they can influence what happens to them, when, in reality, in some cases restrictions are imposed on their human and civil rights and over the control they have over their own lives.

It is not only that service users/survivors may have a particular previously neglected perspective to offer. They also have important new insights to contribute about 'mental health', madness, distress and the responses made to them. Since the 1960s big challenges have emerged to psychiatry and traditional understandings of 'mental health' and 'mental illness'. But initially these mainly came from within psychiatry and related professions themselves; from radical psychiatric thinkers and clinicians: people like Thomas Szasz, the anti-psychiatrists of the 1960s and

1970s, notably R.D. Laing, and critical psychologists and social workers.

More recently, from the 1980s, new critiques began to emerge from service users/survivors themselves. These have much to tell both about being a mental health service user and about the services and systems which define them. Even more important, perhaps, they point to new ways of understanding and addressing madness and distress. That is why this book in the series not only has a contribution to make in terms of telling us more about service users and their understandings of themselves and the world they inhabit, but also in making clear what perpetuates madness and distress and how such phenomena and experiences may best either be prevented or people supported to deal with them as successfully as possible.

This book draws on many people's experiences, ideas and proposals. These are mainly but not exclusively people with first-hand experience of mental distress and mental health services. I have also learned from professionals and practitioners in the field, educators and researchers – and sometimes these have also been people with direct experience as mental health service users. These are people I have got to know, to work with, whose writings and discussions I have learned from. I have also had discussions with some mental health service users specifically as part of writing this book, so it can be informed by their knowledge, experience and understandings.

The aim of this book is to help us make better sense of our and other people's experience as mental health service users and also to be able to play a more active role in society individually and collectively, by building on the strengths of that experience.

The structure of the book

The book is organised in four main parts. The first part offers a picture of how things now are. Chapter 1 sets the scene, introducing the author and considering the experience of being a mental health service user. Chapter 2 offers a broad view of the existing mental health system and what it can feel like to be in it as a service user. The third chapter looks at the language and terminology used in this field, its complexity, and in some cases its cruel and negative purpose and meanings, as well as how mental health service users/survivors have worked to change this.

The second part of the book is concerned with developments that have challenged traditional approaches to mental health. Chapter 4 focuses on the development of the survivor movement and service users' own organisations. Chapter 5 examines some of the serious inequalities that continue to operate in the mental health system and how service users/survivors and their organisations experience and seek to overcome them. In Chapter 6 we see how service users/survivors have worked together to develop their own interpretations of who they are and what has happened to them, to reclaim their identity and act together on the basis of this to bring about change. Chapter 7 focuses on one of the main areas where service users/survivors have felt change is needed. It looks at how mental health issues have tended to be understood. This has largely been through a 'medical model' which many service users find damaging and unhelpful. We look at their efforts and ideas for moving to a more social understanding of 'madness and distress' and how this might help.

Part three of the book looks at what policy and provision might look like if it were based on the ideas, experience and proposals of mental health service users/survivors and was able to cast off its narrowly medicalised inheritance. Chapter 8 sets out the kind of principles and values that might provide the basis for such a transformed survivor-led approach to madness and distress. Chapter 9 explores the kind of support and services that are likely to be helpful in such a survivor-led approach. Chapter 10 sets out a series of helpful routes and commitments to achieving such radical change. It is followed by the fourth part of the book, the Postscript which looks at some of the broader issues that face us living in a 'maddening' world as well as coming back to us as individuals and considering the relationship between the two.

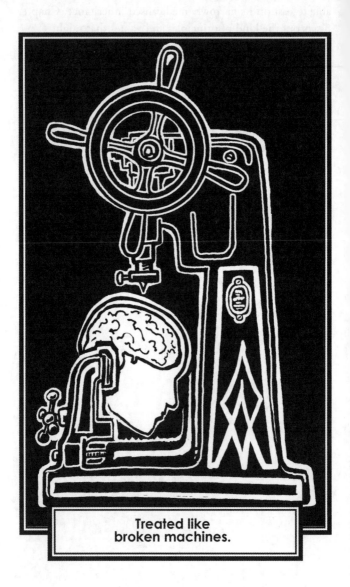

Treated like
broken machines.

Chapter 1
Setting the scene

> I know I get my strength from other service users and on my own probably couldn't do it. So, yes, I think I'm part of a movement that is saying, 'We've got something to say. We could be, we can be useful to society' and that's my feeling.
>
> *Discussion by group of mental health service users/ survivors*

There are few things that can be said with any certainty about our lives as human beings. People's lives are all different. We have different identities, different backgrounds, different circumstances and we may want different things. But one thing does seem to be true. Nobody really wants to become a user of psychiatric or mental health services. How different this is to when we have a physical health problem. Of course no one wants to be physically ill. From childhood we learn to beware the taste of medicine and contact with doctors. But the health service is there for us as a safety net, somewhere to sort out our troubles and be cared for. Very often it can 'make us better'. Who thinks of psychiatric services in this way? I suspect very few, if any of us. Instead they still seem to be the subject of a kind of folk fear – much more like the Victorian poor law workhouse or 'lunatic asylum' than the local GP or modern hospital. We don't see them as places where we will 'get better', but rather somewhere to keep away from. Psychiatric services are something we hope never to have close-up dealings with, least of all for ourselves. For those of us who directly encounter such services, it can feel more like being treated as a broken machine than gaining support, understanding and care.

I remember one afternoon, after collapsing in the street with a panic attack, huddled against a shop window, frightened to move, and then with help, managing to make my way to the health centre to get an emergency appointment with the GP. I didn't know what was happening to me. I was terrified. When I got there, the bureaucracy swung into action. I was told to take a seat. I sat worried and fearful. The doctor walked through the surgery, empty apart from me. He had been my doctor for some time. He walked past me without even looking in my direction. Some time passed before he called me in and I remember no helpful guidance from that consultation. That memory typified for me how the system seemed to see people with mental health problems. It also highlighted for me the difference between bringing a physical and a mental problem to the doctors.

I have often said that I wouldn't wish my experience of mental distress on anyone, except perhaps my worst enemy. I certainly wouldn't suggest it as a route to understanding and enlightenment. I can never get sentimental about my experience of distress or the psychiatric system. A quick think brings it all back into sharp and sometimes nasty relief. But having said that, having had to have that experience and having worked my way through it, I certainly don't wish now that it had never happened to me. I do think I have gained a better understanding of myself and other people as a result. I am proud of what I have overcome and achieved. I am particularly grateful for the path it has helped set me on and for the many other people with shared and similar experience that I have got to know as a result. On balance, I believe the positive outcomes have greatly outweighed the negative ones. I suspect this may be different for many other people, especially those who have not found the support and enlightenment I have been fortunate enough to encounter. Of course, given the choice, I'd far rather it hadn't happened to me, far rather I had found other gentler means of self-discovery and career guidance! But from talking to many others I don't think my experience is unusual or the insights I have gained rare or unique.

Why am I starting by saying all this? Because I believe that in our society, and indeed in many others, we are powerfully discouraged from talking about any experience we have of distress or letting other people know of any psychiatric experience we may have had. Many dread having to turn to such services. I know first-hand of one person who, faced with this prospect, decided to and succeeded in killing himself. He is far from an isolated instance. Many people are left on their own, with secrets and difficulties that are difficult to deal with and which can overshadow their lives and their relationships.

I am a determinedly 'out' mental health service user. I don't want people not to know about my experience. This isn't about flaunting what's happened to me, making it the be-all and end-all of who I am. Rather it is about being honest and open. To be truthful, I couldn't cope not being open. I realised that some time ago and it is why I made my personal choice. I don't want people to be hinting at things behind my back. I don't want my experience to be used or seen as some kind of vulnerability. This is how I can best cope with what happened to me. Each person will have their own way of dealing with these things. Some may want to keep them to themselves and as far as I am concerned that is fine. I have friends and colleagues for whom that is the case and I respect and understand their position. Sometimes it is wisest because of prejudices and power inequalities to be quiet about who we are. But if this book and similar initiatives help one person to feel less guilty or ashamed about themselves, work through what has happened to them, feel they don't have to have secrets unless they want to and get to grips better with demons they may have had, then in my mind, it has been worthwhile.

My background

One of the purposes of this book is to connect the political and the personal; the policies and practices of 'mental health' and psychiatry and the experience of being on the receiving end of them. Because of this, it seems especially important to start by saying a little about who I am and where I am coming from, so the reader can make better sense of what I say. I used statutory mental health services over a period of 12 years. I am no longer using them, but never assume that the need might not arise again. I don't feel that distress, mental health issues, call them what you will, are a thing of the past as far as I am concerned, but rather that I am currently managing to deal with them. I know many people for whom this is true, as well as others who think of their difficulties as in the past and refer to themselves as 'former patients' or ex-mental health service users, or perhaps don't even think of it. One of the key lessons to learn in this field is that we are all truly different. We may gain understanding from each other, but no one should assume that we are all the same; that we react the same, experience the same and that the same things work for us. Being a mental health service user, in both positive and difficult senses, really is about difference and the fact

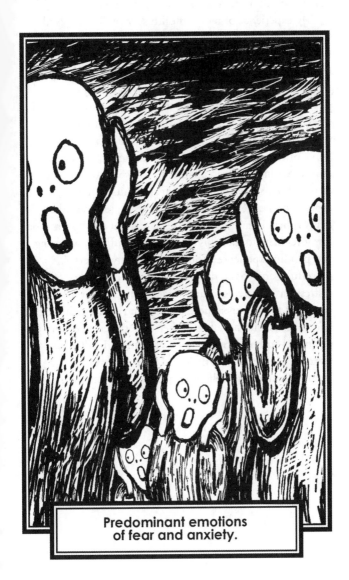

Predominant emotions
of fear and anxiety.

that we are all of us as human beings different.

My experience of mental health services has involved being an inpatient and an outpatient of a psychiatric hospital, seeing psychiatrists and getting long-term support from a psychologist. It has included 'drug therapy', as well as the involvement of many professionals including physiotherapists, occupational therapists, nurses and social workers. It has involved group therapy and art therapy, as well as physical exercise, relaxation and breathing exercises. Some of these interventions have been helpful, others the opposite. I haven't been admitted to hospital under section or used forensic services, so there are limits to my experience. As well as using mental health services, like many others I have lived long term – about eight years – on low level benefits and this for me was a difficult, worrying and painful experience. The fear of poverty lingers powerfully and frighteningly for me. My experience of distress has mostly been unpleasant. The predominant emotions I have experienced are fear and anxiety, although I know others who have found their experience revelatory and positive. I still have better and worse times. I still don't always understand sensations and feelings that I have. I learn more about myself and my distress all the time.

Chapter 2
The psychiatric system

> Power, not illness or treatment, is what the system is all
> about. It is power that usually is not spoken about.[1]
> *Judi Chamberlin*

The first fact that needs to be acknowledged is that the
psychiatric system in a Western society like the UK is large
and complex. If the issue of 'mental health' is sometimes
presented in terms of something strange – a few 'weirdos'
out there – far distant from the rest of 'us', the reality is that
the system exists on an industrial scale. Once there were
enormous rural walled institutions, sometimes with many
hundreds – even thousands – of inmates, which were the
equivalent of villages or local urban communities. They had
their own laundries, shops, workshops, farms, gardens and
food production, libraries, newsletters, power stations,
medical centres, dispensaries, living quarters and staff
residences. Frequently they even had their own chapels and
mortuaries. The modern history of mental health services
has been of the run-down of such institutions.

However, this does not mean that such a wide range of
services and functions no longer exists. Arguably, there are
now more. Nor does it mean that mental health service
users/survivors aren't still segregated and separated from
other people and lumped together with people seen as the
same. There are still psychiatric hospitals and acute inpatient
wards. There are medium secure units and special hospitals

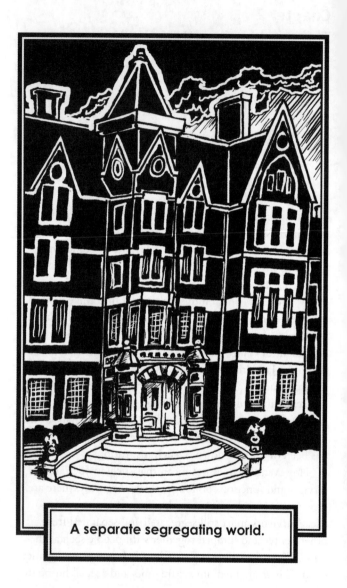

A separate segregating world.

like Rampton and Broadmoor. There are criminal justice diversion schemes. There are day centres, day hospitals, sheltered workshops, employment schemes, crisis, multi-disciplinary mental health and 'assertive outreach' teams, befrienders and volunteers, supported housing, hostels and sheltered housing schemes. There are arts projects, gardening projects, drop-in centres, 'out-of-hours' services, therapeutic communities, helplines and social enterprises. There is almost a parallel universe of provision for people as mental health service users. There are also many mental health service users located in other services, notably in the prison system (now often seen as serving the same institutional role as the old psychiatric hospitals), in provision for homeless people and in related services for people with alcohol and drug problems.

It is important to stress the scale, diversity and complexity of the psychiatric system, with its many different services and its wide range of professions, with different traditions, status and cultures. However much stigma still surrounds the mental health system and the problems that lead people to it, it can no longer truly be seen as an isolated distant world, many miles away from us, separated by high walls and locked doors. The mental health services are now essentially a large locally based system, near where we live, often closely situated alongside other health services and just a referral away from our GP. We may walk past services and facilities each day, perhaps unaware that they are part of this vast parallel world.

Yet the general feeling about the mental health system is negative, however much it has moved on from its institutionally based 19th-century origins. This is not just a folk fear that arises out of ignorance and misunderstanding from people who have never had contact with it and only know it from myth and media. It is a commonly held view among mental health service users themselves, based on their own first-hand experience.

What it can feel like

This is how a long-term survivor friend of mine put it at the time of one admission when he had been very depressed. 'Dave', as I'll call him, had been labelled as a schizophrenic, manic depressive, having personality disorder and much more. This was a time when he felt very down. He said:

I felt suicidal, rubbish, nothing, useless. What I wanted was somewhere safe, somewhere where I'd be OK – sanctuary, asylum ... First they put me in the psychiatric ward of the general hospital. That was OK. Then quite quickly I was sent on to the local psychiatric hospital. It's a big, Victorian institution. [When you speak to Dave on the patient's phone, you can hear the long corridor echoing as people walk along it.] It's not safe. I didn't want to take things like my radio in case they were stolen. The food is rubbish.

There are some good things. Other patients are a positive. The nurses are not too bad this time. Some are OK. They'll talk, but it's five minutes and then they've got to be doing something else, seeing someone else. It's the way it always is. Not enough of them.

But when they say to me, 'you'll come through', are they saying that to me specifically? Do they mean it, or is it just what they say to patients generally? I can see them watching me to make sure I don't do anything, don't hurt myself. I have been 'specialed'. That means they follow you round, but it feels more like it's to protect them than me. There have been more [spending] cuts, even less time seeing the psychiatrists, fewer nurses, less resources and activities.

Nothing really nasty has happened this time. I haven't had or seen any forced medication, verbal or physical abuse.

I met with a small group of mental health service users as part of the process of writing this book in order to include their views. They expressed similar concerns and worries about mental health services. They focused particularly on their experience of inpatient services.

I find that being in the psychiatric hospital is as painful as it has always been. [General agreement]

... you are given full medication and shelter, but it's all you are given ... I feel that there is no psychological input. It's too much based on your medication ... It feels like a prison.

Yes, I saw a psychiatrist once every two weeks or so ... But I didn't feel it was a space in which I could really voice my feelings. It was like a sitting in judgement situation. It didn't feel a friendly atmosphere. I found the OT [occupational therapy] department helpful. I almost consider it as something aside from life in the ward ... The ward, I think it's as dreadful as it's always been ... Because you're not taken care of as an individual. It is as if the fact that you are distressed – in distress – is not considered. You might find the occasional good nurse ... but that's as far as it goes ... Nobody's interested in you and you need so much to talk to someone and ... just that opportunity was never given to me.

Things have improved ... Now you get your own room. In those days [1980s] you slept in a dormitory. You had no privacy.

17

[But] the wards [there] are still very boring places ... You don't get enough stimulation ... A lot of people will still say that the nurses don't talk to you. They're always in the office filling in forms ... They have introduced something called 'protective time' when staff are supposed to speak to you.

There's a growing number of people with 'dual diagnosis' now (people using illegal drugs as well as having other diagnoses attached to them) ... people with drugs, alcohol and solvent abuse ... and they are much more security conscious. Video cameras for the staff to look at, at the entrances to the wards ... I think it has changed for the worse ... They're bringing in police with sniffer dogs at times, to see that something hasn't been brought in.

This reflects much wider comments and experience. A picture emerges from mental health service users/survivors of a psychiatric system which can feel frightening and strange. There can be long delays in accessing services and getting the kind of support people want. Women are still being placed in mixed wards where they feel unsafe, despite government commitment to put an end to them. The quality of acute wards continues to be highlighted in official reports as inadequate. There is a strong backlog of evidence that black and minority ethnic service users face discrimination in mental health services and are more likely to receive controlling than valued provision. Service users can be put at risk from other patients who are aggressive, confused, frightened or using non-prescription drugs, without adequate staff control or supervision. Ward staff are still often poorly trained and sometimes unhelpful, abusive and aggressive. Often they retreat to their offices, rather than being available to help. There are additional problems of communication in wards where English is not the first language of many staff. Shortage of services, resulting in an emphasis on 'recovery' and 'throughput', means that service users are can come under constant pressure to move on before they feel ready, when they are able to access supportive housing or services.

Instead of mental health services necessarily being something that can help deal with the difficulties and mental distress that people are experiencing, they can seem like an additional *obstacle* they have to contend with. As 'Dave' said, when he left hospital, not feeling very good, 'It is as if you have both your distress and the hospital to contend with.' So the first requirement for a mental health service user can sometimes be to be able to deal with the psychiatric system itself – at a time in their life when it is probably because they are having difficulties dealing with things that they are there in the first place.

As editors of an Open University reader on mental health matters wrote in 2009:

> Large proportions of service users and survivors who have experienced the mental health services as 'consumers' still come away dissatisfied with the way they have been treated. There are still precious few reports outside the public relations blurbs of corporate organizational literature of people having positive experiences of mental health services.[2]

The mental health or psychiatric system is not only a large one, it is also a complex one, located in different service systems and departments. It includes health, social care, housing, and benefits organisations. This means that service users have to negotiate local authority, NHS, and welfare agencies. Services may be based in the state, voluntary or private sectors. Each can be expected to have its own particular forms, routes in, culture and ways of doing things. Service users can expect to pass and be passed between different agencies, professionals and service providers, each of which does not necessarily know the processes and ways of working of the other. This is anything but a seamless process, with different arrangements for assessment, different cultures and even significantly different understandings of mental health issues. Again service users need to negotiate this, often with little help or guidance, at what might be times of extreme stress and difficulty in their lives.

It is also not only dedicated mental health services that impact on the lives of people experiencing distress and pose problems for them. The first port of call for many is their GP. As has often been observed, the majority of GP consultations relate to emotional and psychological rather than physical problems, yet often mental health service users wish they could bypass their GP because of their lack of expertise and understanding in this area. Mental health service users have to turn to other services which often treat them in different, inferior ways. Well-charted examples include the experience of people who self-harm with accident and emergency services and the inferior help they receive from the NHS for physical health problems documented in the Disability Rights Commission 'formal investigation' into the physical health inequalities experienced by mental health service users.[3] It is also in the context of such other services that issues about the stigma and stereotyping associated with being a mental health service user emerge that can have powerful effects on people's lives and their feelings about themselves.

The dominance of 'diagnosis'

Another key point needs to be made about the psychiatric system. Everything tends to be determined by the diagnostic category in which you are included. This shapes how you are seen, the treatment you receive and the nature of your journey through the system. It may even play a crucial role in whether that treatment is on a compulsory or voluntary basis. It is through diagnostic categorisation that the psychiatric system organises both itself and service users. Diagnosis is the basis for the expertise, specialist knowledge and skills that psychiatrists, the dominant psychiatric system profession, claim. Their role revolves round assessing, categorising, classifying and treating people. Not everyone knows their own diagnosis. Sometimes psychiatrists are reluctant to convey it to service users, but everyone is likely to have a diagnosis attached to them. Many service users find their diagnosis reassuring. They feel it helps them explain and make sense of their feelings and situation. Others reject the labels attached to them.

Diagnosis is far from an exact science. The diagnoses attached to people can change, vary with different psychiatrists and with different ethnic groupings. African-Caribbean young men, for example, have tended to be diagnosed disproportionately as 'psychotic' and 'schizophrenic'. The basis for such diagnostic categorization since 1952 has been the *Diagnostic and Statistical Manual of Mental Disorders* (DSM) which is published by the American Psychiatric Association and provides diagnostic criteria for 'mental disorders'. Now in its fourth edition, the DSM has always been contentious.[4] It is criticised for reflecting dominant values so that for a long time it identified homosexuality as a category of 'disorder' and even now retains the category 'sexual orientation disturbance'.

Over the years it has included an increasing number of diagnostic categories but continues to be adversely criticised for being subjective, unreliable, inconsistent and Eurocentric.

The development of something different

Not surprisingly, for many mental health service users, dealing with their distress and the additional difficulties they can face from being in mental health services takes all their energy and attention. Add to this the fact that all this may be happening at times of isolation, confusion and uncertainty, and few may feel in a position to analyse, let alone challenge what is happening to them. The role of 'mental patient' has long been one constructed in very passive terms with the individual questioned, categorised and 'treated', with minimal opportunities to play an active role in the process or explore what they feel or want. The effect is further to separate and individualise people. Perhaps it is not surprising that a key media image of mental health service users is as people acting strangely and separately in some institutional, hospital or public setting.

Yet despite the scale of the barriers and the difficulties, the late 20th century witnessed the emergence of collective action on the part of mental health service users in the UK and internationally. It is this development which lies at the heart of this book. It is the fruits of this movement that the book is based upon. It is the lessons which the service user movement has taught us that the book seeks to explore and share. Some of the key points that the movement has established are that there is a life during and after madness and distress; that these need to be recognised as part of all our experiences and identities; that people experiencing madness and distress are people too; that mental health service users have human and civil rights that must be respected and that there are different and better ways of engaging with madness and distress than traditional medicalised approaches have suggested.

The mental health service user/survivor movement has both offered us different ways of understanding the experience, concepts and apparatus of 'mental illness' and of being a mental health service user, and also begun a process of developing new experiences, ideas and responses to these phenomena.

We will shortly be examining the origins of the survivor movement, but first more needs to be said about language in this field.

Chapter 3
The language of 'mental health'

> Until there is common agreement on what is meant by
> 'mental illness', there can be no common language for the
> related concepts of patients/service users/survivors/
> consumers, etc. ... Ultimately, different people will
> describe themselves differently, and this is as it should be,
> since our movement stresses the right to self-define.[1]
> *Jan Wallcraft and Mary Nettle*

Language in the context of 'mental health' is a field of
conflict. It is almost impossible to escape this. Even my
opening sentence is contentious because of the baggage that
concepts like 'mental health' carry. It is hardly surprising
that terminology in this field is problematic, given that it
relates to what is widely seen as a stigmatising, spoiled and
devalued identity – using 'mental health services' and being
'mentally ill'.

There is no agreement about terminology in relation to
'mental health service users' and the 'survivor movement'.
This means that whatever terms are used are likely to offend
someone. My aim in the language I have used in this book is
to try to offend as few people as possible and to be
consistent with the values which generally underpin the
collective action of mental health service users/survivors – of
which more later. But we have to be honest and admit that
language continues to be a problem in this field and it can
have a damaging and divisive effect, sending out all kinds of

unhelpful messages. Language also has a particular importance in this field because so often it has been negative and so many negative or pejorative words have been developed to describe it.

Traditional formal language used about mental health service users/survivors has largely been rejected by service user activists. The terms used have either followed from their role in the psychiatric system as *patients*, or been associated with the diagnostic categories in which they have been included. Thus the most commonly used term has been 'patient', or 'psychiatric' or 'mental' patient. Many service users/survivors reject such terms because they feel they emphasise their passivity and frame them narrowly in terms of services which they frequently dislike and reject. People are also described in terms of diagnostic categories as 'schizophrenics', 'manic-depressives' or 'bipolars'. Such labels are frequently experienced as demeaning, reducing people to a set of symptoms, framing them in narrow medical terms. They are especially problematic because the diagnostic categories attached to people frequently change, overlap and do not seem to be consistently applied. Such labels are especially felt to objectify and reduce the people they are attached to. Having said that, when such labels have been attached to people, they sometimes use them of themselves, perhaps because they seem to offer them an explanation or justification for their situation and the difficulties they may experience. As has been said, there is no consensus here!

There is another set of terminology that needs to be touched on. This is the frequently derogatory, stigmatic and abusive language that is used about distress and mental health service users in popular and media discussion. A wide and growing range of such terms continues to be used and developed, which includes words like 'nutter', 'loony', 'nut case', 'mental case', 'mental', 'mentalist', 'psycho', 'community care case' and 'crazy'. Some can be seen as leftovers from previous ages. Others have much more recent origins. They are part of our cultural wallpaper, featuring in TV programmes for both adults and children as terms of ridicule and rejection. They are part of a broader environment of stigma and exclusion which mental health service users routinely encounter and which I will look at more directly elsewhere in this book.

Because the language associated with 'mental health issues' has been seen by survivors as so damaging and discriminatory, from the time that they started to develop their own groups and organisations in the 1980s, they have sought to develop their own alternatives. Two terms have been at the heart of their attempts to describe themselves. These are *survivor* and *service user*. The term *survivor* seems to have had its origins in the pioneering mental health service users' organisation Survivors Speak Out. This talked of people as psychiatric system survivors. The emphasis was placed on people surviving what had happened and been done to them in the psychiatric system. Others talked about mental health and psychiatric survivors, meaning people who were surviving their difficulties and distress. People also began to talk of themselves as psychiatric or mental health service users. This connected with the development of other service user organisations and movements like those of disabled people, people with learning difficulties, those living with HIV/AIDS and older people. It was seen as offering a preferable alternative to the term patient.

However, both these terms, *survivor* and *service user*, have come in for criticism. The term survivor was seen to create confusion with people who had survived domestic or sexual abuse. The term 'user' was again seen as too passive, defining people in terms of services they often did not want to receive. Some people also dislike it because of its association with drug 'user'. Yet these continue to be the two most frequently used terms among service users/ survivors, for all their shortcomings. This is why I use here the term *mental health service user/survivor,* since it probably comes as close as we can get to reflecting the spirit of how people want to identify themselves, even if it has weaknesses of its own. This term seems to cause the least offence. I use it to mean people who currently or in the past have used mental health services or who would be seen as eligible to use them. There is an argument that we are all 'people' first and that it is therefore unhelpful to describe ourselves distinctly as service users or survivors. But this ignores the reality that people with experience of distress and/or of using mental health services are likely to be seen and treated as different. Thus ignoring this denies their experience.

The advent of managerialism and consumerism in public policy has led to an increasing emphasis on terms like *customer* or *consumer.* Many survivor activists reject such terms, particularly since many mental health service users are involuntary users who are subjected to treatment under compulsory section. Mike Lawson, for example, one of the founders of the survivor movement, observed that psychiatric system survivors are 'consumers of mental health services in the same way that rats are consumers of Rentokil'. Other terms like service *refuser* have also been developed by survivors.

Service users have also sought to move beyond prevailing medical models to describe the experiences they have. Thus they have tended to talk much more about 'distress' – emotional and mental distress – than mental health or mental health problems. Some also talk about madness, although some others are uncomfortable with the term. Service users have not only worked to develop their own terminology, they have also sought to reappropriate and reclaim existing language. Thus they have used the terms 'madness' to describe differences and extremes of emotion and perception. They have used the word in a non-pejorative way. This can be seen as part of a broader development, where mental health service users/survivors, like other oppressed groups and minorities, including black and minority ethnic people, women, gay men, lesbians, bisexuals and transsexuals, seek to reclaim oppressive language used against them, particularly in their communication with each other. Thus the emergence of 'Mad Pride', a campaigning and activist organisation committed to challenging the devalued position of mental health service users/survivors.

Chapter 4
The mental health service user/survivor movement

> What underpins this is a drive, a will to see real
> improvement for service users in terms of treatment
> options, of people actively participating in their care, and
> in terms of real social inclusion. I think that for me it has
> become more than a journey of discovery or a healing
> process; it is also now a political engagement, an act of
> citizen participation ...[1]
>
> *Anne-Laure Donskoy*

The modern mental health service user/survivor movement
is a very recent development. Its origins are usually traced to
the mid 1980s. It represents a fundamental watershed in
mental health issues. Yet of course many people, including
many service users, don't know about this movement. This
is hardly surprising, but doesn't make it any less significant.
We live in a world where the storylines of soaps make
headline news, where people who happen to see media stars
in the street think they know them because they are so used
to seeing them in their homes on their television and
computer screens. Yet issues affecting the day-to-day lives of
millions of people tend only to be picked up by the media if
some exceptional problem, tragedy or unusual occurrence is
involved.

People still frequently talk and write about 'the mentally
ill' as though they were a distant separate group of people
very different from the rest of 'us'. Discussion is still often

framed in terms of what can 'we' do about 'them'. Not only does this fly in the face of the facts – it has been well established that very high proportions of people are likely to be affected by 'mental health problems' during the course of their lives – a figure of one in four is often given. But also most of us can expect someone close to us to have such experiences, including what are seen as the most severe and difficult problems of distress. So although the tendency is to frame mental health issues in terms of 'other' people, and later we will look at why this might be, the reality is that they are much more helpfully understood as part of the human condition; something that may affect any one of us, which we can routinely expect to encounter in one way or another in our lives.

This is only the first routine inaccuracy we can expect to encounter over this issue. Another is that there is an active 'we' who are the solution and a passive 'them' who are the problem. It is unlikely that this has ever been true, but certainly over the last 20 to 30 years very visible events have given the lie to it. This is the emergence of mental health service user/survivor organisations and a distinct survivor movement. The development of this movement and these organisations means that mental health service users themselves are playing an active and distinct role in doing something about mental health issues. While this role should not be exaggerated, equally it can no longer be ignored. Mental health service users, their organisations and movement can be seen as a new player in the game, bringing new ideas, knowledge, understandings, proposals and solutions to the table. So mental health service user/survivor is a term now that may not only mean we have experience on the receiving end of mental health/psychiatric services. It is now also, as will be discussed in more detail in the next chapter, a political identity, meaning that people actively engage over these issues from their experience and role in relation to the psychiatric system.

It is this development of the survivor movement and its implications for individual mental health service users/ survivors and mental health policy and practice that we want to look at in this part of the book.

Peter Campbell, a founding member of the survivors' movement, has written of its development:

> Since 1980 the mental health system in the United Kingdom (UK) has changed dramatically. While the main types of care and treatment provided by mental health services have changed little, the location of services and mechanisms of delivery have undergone significant alteration. Simultaneously and partly as a direct result of these transformations, those diagnosed as mentally ill, the current and former mental patients, have become more visible and vocal within society and in the corridors of power. Government seeks their views. The service provider is obliged to consult with them.[2]

Peter Campbell identifies much earlier examples of activism and protests by 'mad persons' from the seventeenth century onwards. However, he dates the modern UK survivor movement from the mid 1980s and traces its origins to earlier mental patient groups from the beginning of the 1970s and acknowledges the support it gained from radical mental health professionals.[3] He also makes the important point that survivors like him were more able to get engaged in this way as services became more community based from the 1960s, rather than being segregated long term within institutions. There has also been a developing two-way traffic of ideas and action between the UK survivor movement and its equivalents in European countries and

North America. A worldwide movement now exists. There are worldwide, European, national, regional and local organisations and groups of mental health service users/ survivors. As Peter Campbell notes, over an amazingly short period we have gone from a situation in the UK where less than a dozen independent user/survivor-led action groups existed to one today where numbers are probably at least in the high hundreds, although it is difficult to be precise, since groups and organisations tend to come and go. [4]

What is also important about the survivor movement is that a very wide range of people with experience of mental health services have been involved in its founding and development. This includes people who had spent a long time in psychiatric hospitals, people much of whose lives had been spent in and out of such hospitals, people identified as having the most serious or severe diagnoses, who had tried to kill themselves, who had ongoing problems of depression, self-harm and eating distress. It has also included people who have been politically active as well as others who have never got involved before, people from many different black and ethnic communities, men and women, older and younger people, lesbians, gay, bisexual and transgender people as well as heterosexuals.

As Peter Campbell also helpfully makes clear, there is not one single position or view among people who are active in service user/survivor organisations and the survivor movement. They may focus on different issues, have different priorities and see things in different terms.[5] But they have one thing in common, which unites them and on which they tend to be agreed. All start from having personal experience of mental distress, madness and/or using mental health services. It is this direct experience, or as it is sometimes called 'experiential knowledge', which they have in common and which is their unifying force.

The mental health service user/survivor movement has not emerged in isolation. First it needs to be understood in terms of the development of other movements of health, welfare and social care service users. These include movements of disabled people, people with learning difficulties, older people and people living with HIV/AIDS. The earliest established and best known of these movements is the disabled people's movement, which began to establish itself in the UK and internationally in the 1970s. While there are differences in the history, nature and objectives of each of these movements, they have some important concerns in common. All attach great importance to:

- the right of service users to speak for themselves
- their equal worth as human beings with other people
- the importance of their human and civil rights and needs being met

These service user movements also see links between themselves and the 'new social movements' that emerged internationally particularly from the 1960s and 1970s, including the black civil rights movement, the women's movement, the gay men, lesbians, bisexuals and transgender movement and the older people's/grey power movement. What distinguishes these movements is that they have grown out of the sense of oppression and discrimination felt by the groups who have established them. They represent determined efforts to speak and act on their own behalf – to 'self-organise' – and develop aims, ideas, ways of working and cultures of their own to achieve their own self-defined goals.[6,7] These are movements which are based on identity and people's efforts to define their own identity. Identity is a key issue in relation to mental health service users/survivors and we will return to it shortly.

These movements represented a new politics that is not confined narrowly to people's material situation or class and economic relations – important though these are. They were also linked with concerns about broader issues, like the environment, peace and nuclear weapons. All have been concerned with developing new approaches to involvement, diversity and the extension of democracy beyond formal and bureaucratic structures and approaches. Each has developed its own culture or cultures. The same has been true for service user movements. They have been more than just organisationally based. To enable the involvement of people who traditionally had often been excluded from political and collective involvement, all have highlighted the development of new ways of organising, new ways of doing things, new kinds of culture and arts, the development of new ideas and different forms of expression.

Empowerment

Some people see service user movements like the survivor movement as 'new social movements'; others as liberatory movements and there has been much academic discussion about this. Whichever interpretation is placed upon them, however, there seem to be two important and interrelated things that such movements do. These are:

1. Provide opportunities for people to get a better understanding of themselves and gain personal and practical skills

2. Work together to achieve broader political and social change

Key commentators of these movements, like Mike Oliver of the disabled people's movement, have stressed that working

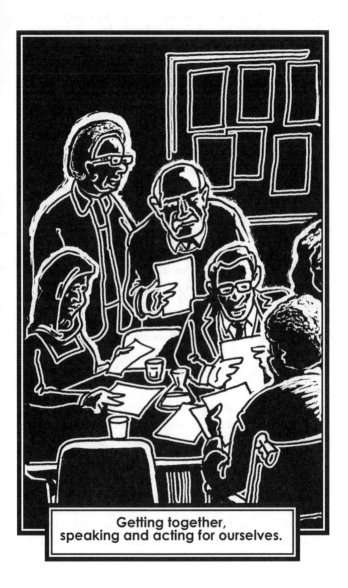

Getting together,
speaking and acting for ourselves.

35

together or taking 'collective action' is the best route to achieving both of these. In our society, there is a lot of emphasis on 'self-help' books and how people can turn their lives round and become more assertive or 'successful' by doing things individually, on their own.[8] A crucial principle of such movements, including the survivor movement, is that we are much more likely to achieve such change – in ourselves and beyond, by getting together with other people. Over the last 50 years or so a new concept has developed which embodies this view. It is called *empowerment*. Although the term is often used in vague and unclear ways and has lost some of its power and value as a result, it is still very helpful. First popularised by the Black Civil Rights movement in the USA, what it highlights is that making social and political change is inseparable from making personal change. One is unlikely to happen without the other. So empowerment as a radical idea is concerned with:

- making change within ourselves
- working together from this position to make broader societal change[9]

Both are essential and the belief is that if political change is truly to be inclusive and democratic, then we will all need to be involved in the process and a process of growth and development will also need to take place within each of us.

Service user/survivor organisations

There are many different kinds of service user/survivor organisations, big and small, doing different things. Some focus particularly on offering mutual aid and support, others are more concerned with campaigning and activism, while others are concerned with both. Both aims are valued in service user organisations, as are the interrelations between them. Some organisations are democratically constituted, with written constitutions, others are more informal. Some are closely bound up with services and work to help people who are currently in such services and may owe their origins to enthusiastic professionals who helped initiate them. Others provide services themselves. Some are closely linked with traditional charitable organisations, others are more determinedly independent. Some longstanding voluntary organisations, like Mind and Together, have user groups or user sections. There are networks, user groups and organisations for people with particular experiences and diagnoses, for example, people who hear voices, who self-harm or are identified as having 'bipolar disorder' or 'schizophrenia'. Others are organised around issues of difference, for example, for and of black and minority ethnic mental health service users or lesbians. There are user groups operating in hospitals and services, as well as in communities and linked with day and other services.

The many local organisations and groups of mental health service users/survivors can be seen as the movement's lifeblood. They can take many forms, providing a base both for activism and mutual support. As Mary Nettle, longstanding survivor activist and researcher, says:

> The user/survivor movement cannot exist without a place for people to meet and swop experiences; this often starts with being an inpatient in hospital and carries on outside hospital settings often run by well meaning voluntary organisations which often have the same attitudes as are found in hospital. However they can be a catalyst for people who want more than just a cup of tea and a chat and it can then become a safe place to discuss what could

be better about the mental health system locally. In order
to do this, information is shared and a group may be
formed. People may want to know more and find out or
are told about national user/survivor groups. Some are safe
like Mindlink within Mind, others more challenging such as
the late-lamented Survivors Speak Out. People can then
begin to spread their wings but in my view need to have
support to be just a user/survivor at grassroots level.

While a number of national organisations of mental health
service users/survivors have been established, perhaps most
significantly, Survivors Speak Out and the United Kingdom
Advocacy Network (UKAN), these have tended to face
particular problems of funding, security and in some cases
credibility, as Peter Campbell has also suggested.[10] While of
course in terms of overall numbers of people with
experience of distress or using mental health services, the
numbers involved in service user organisations can be seen
as quite small (and although there are no accurate figures,
they certainly number in the thousands), this is an
unprecedented development – at both personal and political
levels. These are people who in the past would neither have
had the opportunity, or in all likelihood ever have expected
to be actively involved alongside other people with similar
experience. By doing so they challenge both other people's
and their own expectations of themselves. This says a lot
about what mental health service users/survivors are capable
of – given the chance. In the next section we will look more
closely at the status and identity of mental health service
users/survivors, which highlights even more the great leap
forward this development of collective action and the
survivor movement represents.

Earlier we heard from Mary Nettle, a survivor activist
and researcher. She was also until recently the Chair of the

European Network of (ex) Users and Survivors of Psychiatry (ENUSP). As she makes clear, while many barriers remain, survivors and their movement are now operating on an international scale as well as starting with the strength of their grassroots organisations:

> It is possible to move from grassroots to national to European and international within the user/survivor movement more easily than you would think. All it needs is the will to want to look further than your own situation and the support to see that it is possible. Resources are always an issue as user survivors are amongst the poorest members of society, and a broadband Internet connection in your own home now makes communication and knowledge exchange so much easier. The reality of living with a psychiatric label is what binds us together despite cultural and legal differences. The work on the UN Convention of Rights of People with Disabilities has led to a treaty which will make a difference to our lives as user/ survivors when we are informed by our peers in the international movement WNUSP (World Network of (ex) Users and Survivors of Psychiatry) and backed up at the European level by ENUSP (European Network of (ex) Users and Survivors of Psychiatry). Both organisations struggle for resources and rely on voluntary effort and some membership fees to exist. Both manage to get people together for occasional general assemblies to ensure that they are more than just a virtual body joined by the Internet.

Chapter 5
Mental health services and inequality

Black service users/survivors think that there is an emerging Black movement but it is very fragmented at the moment. There is a need for groups to come together to support and sustain one another and some evidence shows this is beginning to happen. But the people we spoke to find they are often not supported by larger organisations that could help them with funding and other resources, and Black service users/survivors who are working hard to raise awareness often end up feeling unheard, unvalued and exhausted.[1]

Jan Wallcraft, Jim Read and Angela Sweeney

Madness, mental distress and using mental health services tend not to be valued in Western societies like the UK. Instead we know that we can expect the opposite kind of response. As with other aspects of life, there have been some recent attempts to associate mental health problems more positively with celebrity. But as one mental health service user recently wrote:

Bipolar disorder is often 'glamorised' these days by its association with creative types such as Stephen Fry, but my own experience of the illness is far from that.[2]

Although we hear of other societies where madness and distress are valued and celebrated, it is difficult to come across examples of this in modern Western societies. Of course, sometimes issues associated with distress and madness, like hearing voices, self-harm or suicide, are highly regarded, but in those cases they tend to be linked with other situations, qualities or values which lead to them being given a value that would not ordinarily be extended to mental health service users/survivors. Such phenomena, like seeing visions and hearing voices are, for example, associated with many religions and expressions of spirituality, from Christian saints to Shamanism.

Links between 'mental health problems' and inequality are well established.[3] Thus, not only can people generally expect to be seen in a negative light if they are associated with 'mental health problems'. Groups already experiencing discrimination and oppression also tend to run more risk of being linked with such a negative status and to be treated worse if and when they are. In this way, the mental health system and madness and distress have been strongly linked with inequality and the devaluing of difference. Indeed the psychiatric system can be seen as one which has worked to reinforce and enforce conformity and to undermine and reject diversity. Thus groups which face material and social disadvantage and discrimination in society may be more likely to come the way of the psychiatric system and then face more difficult experiences if they do.

This seems to happen in relation to all forms of difference, including diversity in terms of gender, sexuality, ethnicity, belief, class, age, disability, culture and so on.[4,5] A sad reality of the psychiatric system seems to be that it reflects and reinforces broader discriminations, rather than challenging them. One less often mentioned is that concerning age. Young people seem particularly poorly served by mental health services, while older people appear to be at especial risk of receiving inferior, poor quality services and support, if they receive any. Yet older people are a group with high rates of organic mental illness in the form of dementia.

We will look at two areas of discrimination in particular, but this should not be taken to mean that problems are unique or exceptional to these cases.

Sexuality

Linda McFarlane, for example, in a qualitative study of lesbians, gay men and bisexuals in mental health services concluded that while negative responses to their sexuality had an impact on the mental health of most participants, they did not have equal access to mental health services, the quality of the response to them was patchy, lack of safety was an urgent issue, discriminatory attitudes were pervasive and mainstream services needed 'vast improvement'. She evidenced high levels of homophobia within the mental health services, showing how this further exacerbated the distress experienced by users.[6]

Patsy Staddon identifies as a mental health service user/survivor and has long-term experience of homelessness and using alcohol. She is now a user researcher and from her experience and research highlights the problems facing lesbians in this context:

> Most lesbians I have spoken to attempt to conceal their sexual identity in treatment, so it is not well documented although Busfield has pointed out that 'severe mental health problems may themselves result from the infringement of human rights'.[7] Depression and anxiety are believed to be common among lesbians and caused by homophobia[8] (see also the Alcohol Concern website, www.alcoholconcern.org.uk). Bent and McGilvy[9] produced

42

evidence that such depression is likely to result from feeling different, fearing the consequences of sexual orientation becoming known, either while a child or as an adult in the workplace, and feeling unable to share personal details such as loss of a partner. Lesbians without good support are particularly likely to kill themselves, due to depression and isolation.[10] These issues were also evidenced in my own research. As I have written:

> Being a member of a minority is stressful and lesbians more than heterosexual women tend to feel the ill effects of a value system based on a heteronormativity. This is especially true for those who have felt unable to live open lives. Homophobia creates depression, a major factor among women who misuse alcohol (Kendler et al., 1993). Lesbians can become unhappy and depressed because of their families' incomprehension of their lesbianism, their inability to share in the lives of heterosexual workmates and their being ignored by the health providers and educators. If the lesbian scene is not for them, they may experience loneliness. For them, alcohol can be exciting and pleasurable: 'You get what you need from drugs', (respondent quoted in Raine, 2001, p. 23). It would not be surprising if some lesbians abuse alcohol and feel unable to control their alcohol intake. Some research indicates that stigma, alienation, discrimination, and the cultural importance of bars place lesbians more at risk of developing problems with alcohol than heterosexual women (Rule, 2003). Other research supports the idea that lesbian drinking is more problematic than that of heterosexual women (Jaffe et. al., 2000).[11]

Ethnicity and 'race'

The treatment of black people and members of minority ethnic groups in the psychiatric system mirrors and makes worse the wider discriminations which they face. African-Caribbean and African people, for example, are over-represented in psychiatric institutions. They are most likely (along with Irish people) to be kept in locked wards, to be given higher does of potentially hazardous medication than other groups and are more likely than other ethnic groups to be diagnosed with schizophrenia. African-Caribbean people, particularly young men, are more likely to be referred to mental health services by the criminal justice system than by GPs or social services, to be 'treated' with physical rather than talking therapies and admitted to secure services. They are over-represented in special hospitals, medium secure units and prisons. The evidence continues to show that mental health services are not adequately meeting the needs of black and minority ethnic (BME) communities because they are not sufficiently sensitive or responsive to the diversity of culture, needs and experience and that these groups have little confidence in them. While the government has not accepted this, concerns have been expressed at the highest levels that mental health services are 'institutionally racist'.

Patricia Chambers, a service user/survivor and researcher and activist who is currently working as a project manager in mental health for a BME Health organisation, says:

> Being black and in the psychiatric system is bad for your mental health. You're not taken as seriously having a problem until the situation has escalated to the stage where you've hurt yourself or someone else. Quite often the only way to survive the mental health system is to 'do

your own thing' within it and hope you don't get caught. We are coming into the system at three times the rate of other racial groups. We are more likely to be restrained when in the system then any other racial group and more likely to be given medication rather than talking therapy and we are making up the majority of patients on the locked and secure wards and the average stay on the secure wards is ten years and the cherry on the top of the cake is that you can also lose your life in the mental health system. Something that if you're black you're very much aware of. Where are the white David 'Rocky' Bennetts or Orville Blackwoods? The picture is very bleak and yet we are expected to entrust our precious brains, intellect and spirit to a system that is failing us. And we know it.

Refugees and asylum seekers are a particularly vulnerable group because of the trauma and loss they have frequently experienced. Their situation can be expected to worsen as their access to benefits and services is further restricted and media campaigns and aggressive political policies increase the stigma and hostility that they face. Black people and minority ethnic groups are still under-represented in service user/survivor groups and organisations. While they have established their own local and national self-help and self-advocacy organisations, these often face particular difficulties maintaining their independence and securing and keeping funding.[12,13]

Jenny Morris, writing from a disability perspective, casts helpful light on how the oppressive nature of mental health services can be expected to interact with other inequalities and discriminations:

As far as the question of whether it is 'gender or disability', or indeed 'race or sexuality' which are the more important determinants of experience, I don't find this way of looking at our lives very helpful either. I think this is partly because our experiences are not fragmented into analytical categories. When Ayesha Vernon interviewed other Black and ethnic minority women, she found that 'Disabled Black and ethnic minority women experience a multiplicity of barriers resulting from the combination of disability or gender which determine their experiences, as one of them put it, "it happens singularly, plurally and multiply, and it's the totality that counts at the end of the day. You are completely thought of as inferior because you are all three things."'[14]

This is likely to apply equally for mental health service users/survivors where the discriminatory effects of such provision operate in complex interaction with other broader inequalities and discriminations in society, imposing negative identities on people and reinforcing stigma and negative stereotypes. This brings us to our next key concern: how the survivors' movement has helped people challenge the negative identities imposed upon them as users of mental health services.

Chapter 6
Issues of identity

> My 'recovery' from persistent suicidal feelings came about
> through spiritual self-enquiry after all the psycho-
> medications and talking therapies had failed and
> sometimes made things worse. Following this spirit of
> enquiry, it now seems fairly natural, (though blessed with
> much good luck) that before long I found myself doing a
> doctorate looking into the first-person perspective on
> suicidality. Doing a doctorate has been its own
> extraordinary journey and adventure.[1]
> *David Webb*

We have seen how using mental health services can add to
your difficulties and be treated as something negative. In
societies like ours, being a mental health service user has
long been what sociologists call having a 'spoiled identity'.
Few would want to identify as having used mental health
services. It is something most people want to keep to
themselves. They can expect others to be put off them if
they find out. Such a status is likely to have a seriously
damaging effect on anyone's self-image, hopes and life
chances.

However, this has begun to change fundamentally. I am
not talking here about the efforts that are more broadly
being made to challenge negative public views of mental
health service users. I am referring specifically to the efforts
of service users *themselves*, particularly over the last 20 or so

years, to rethink who they are – to 'reclaim' their identity. Of course, we can guess that over the years, many people experiencing madness, distress and the psychiatric system have tried to make sense of what is happening to them and have developed their own understandings and interpretations of their feelings and emotions. There is a large and influential literature of such writings by and about people with such experience, ranging from Sylvia Plath's *The Bell Jar*, to Ken Kesey's *One Flew Over the Cuckoo's Nest*. The development of the survivors' movement and the opportunities it has provided for people to come together in groups and organisations, however, has been central in enabling mental health service users/survivors to reflect on and reassess their identity and to challenge dominant versions and accounts of it.

Being a mental health service user: Who are we talking about

While it may in popular imagination conjure up some very rigid stereotypes, the identity of 'mental health service user' actually embraces a very wide range of people, circumstances and experiences. Talk to people involved in a service user organisation or group and you can expect to meet a wide range of mental health service users. They are likely to include people who have spent years in psychiatric hospitals, who have had numerous 'breakdowns', been subject to compulsory sections, who have spent much of their life living on medication and poverty-level benefits. Expect them to include people in employment as well as people who have found the labour market too difficult to work in, people who are or have been homeless, or in the prison system, are included as having 'severe and enduring mental illness' and have had every kind of psychiatric diagnostic label attached to them. There will be people who fit hostile media stereotypes of 'loner' because of their isolation and breakdown of relationships, as well as people living with partners and families, bringing up children and supporting others. There will also be service users who have made every effort to keep out of the system as best they can for years, but for whom it still looms large in their lives because of their fears of coming into contact with it again.

Who are we?

Each of us at some point or points in our life is likely to think, 'who am I?' It is one of the big questions human beings ask. Why am I here? What is the meaning of life? Where do we all come from and where are we heading? We may think about our identity in relation to our family and others, in relation to the past or with hopes and plans for the future. People sometimes talk about 'reinventing' themselves. Each of us has fixed elements making up our identity: for example, the period in which we live, our gender, ethnicity, country of origin. But as well as these objective realities, there are also all the subjective issues of how we see ourselves and indeed how others see us. We hear of famous and beautiful people who have always been unhappy with their looks.

When we experience distress, a breakdown or 'mental health problem', it can be a catastrophic, shattering and unprecedented experience. It can be difficult to think it through carefully, to try and take stock and reflect. That's certainly how it was for me! We may be in turmoil. We may have little to go on. It's quite likely that if anybody else we know has had similar things happen to them, they won't have talked about them. If we turn for help to popular discussions of madness or distress, or what the 'experts' tell us, our anxieties may be increased rather than reduced. For most of us, having a 'mental health problem' is something cataclysmic to our selves and we may have little equipment to deal with it. Given this, it is not surprising that many mental health service users are glad to have a diagnostic label attached to them, which at least suggests that their experience is not unique and unprecedented, even if such labelling can be frightening and stigmatising. The likelihood is that we will 'internalise' prevailing views of 'people like us'. We will see ourselves as others see us: 'ill', 'sick', 'non-functioning', devalued and different. Superimposing this mindset on all the issues that may go with our experience of distress is only likely to make it more difficult for us to deal with and to escape assumptions and preconceptions about us and our possible future.

Identity: Traditional approaches

For a long time, people who use psychiatric or mental health services have been talked about as a distinct and separate group. This has reflected their segregation and separation in society. While terms have changed, this has been a constant. So we have had 'lunatics', 'the insane', 'the mentally disordered', 'the mentally ill' and 'people with mental health problems'. The penultimate two terms are still frequently used. Labels have become more euphemistic, but they denote the same devalued category. Such terms have been linked with the language, institutions and systems by which people have been understood and defined. Talk of people as 'neurotic' and 'psychotic' has entered vernacular language. People have also commonly been described according to the diagnostic labels which are attached to them, for example, as 'schizophrenic', 'bipolar', 'manic depressive' and so on. As we have said it is difficult to avoid internalising these identities and seeing yourself in these terms too. We can be a parent, a partner, husband, wife, worker and much more. But suddenly it can all be reduced to being a mental health service user. This can take over from other things and become people's *defining* identity.

However, the emergence of the survivor movement and survivor organisations has at last given people the chance to think again about their situation and their identity – in association with others who have gone through similar experiences.

Defining our own identities

Getting together in groups provides a chance for service users to have safe discussions with others who have been through similar situations, without any sense of being judged, without having to worry what others will think of them, without the assumption that they must be 'mad' or 'weird' or 'strange'. It can make it possible for them for the first time to talk freely and openly about what they have been through. It no longer has to seem like it's 'all their own fault', or that it denotes there is 'something wrong with them'. People can at last be in a position and feel able to analyse the system that has constantly analysed them. Its analysis of them, whatever its intention, has too often seemed condemnatory. It has felt judgemental, constantly reinforcing views of them as defective and inferior. Ironically, although the psychiatric system has been strong on such analysis, this has not often served as the starting point for effective intervention and improvement. It might offer a powerful system of analysis – one which can frequently feel crushing to those included within it – but the evidence is that this has not necessarily provided the basis for valued, reliable and effective 'treatments'. Modern physical medicine by contrast has been characterised by its increasing ability at least to ameliorate and sometimes to cure conditions that originally were seen as irrevocable and fatal, from cancer and tuberculosis, to HIV and childhood leukaemia.

The emergence of the survivors' movement has made it possible for service users to gain different understandings of themselves and place different interpretations on their circumstances and experience. Even where this does not happen, it has made it possible to gain hope and raised expectations through seeing what other service users in similar circumstances have managed to do. It has truly given people the chance to rethink in positive terms who they are and what they might be.

This doesn't mean that all mental health service users/ survivors will see themselves the same or in the same way. Not everyone will necessarily feel pride in being mad, or want to attach such a word to themselves. Some of us may still feel weighed down and restricted by our experience of madness or distress. Imposing orthodoxy on how we see ourselves is unlikely to be any more helpful than having other people do the same thing to us. What does become more possible is for us not to have to blame ourselves for our situation or see it solely in terms of something wrong with us or that we have done wrong. It makes it possible to recognise the broader relations of such experience and that it neither invalidates us as people in our own right or means that achievements, successes and indeed happiness will inevitably be beyond any of us and pass us by.

Identity politics

Such a reconception of who we are – our identity – and the recognition that we are part of something bigger and

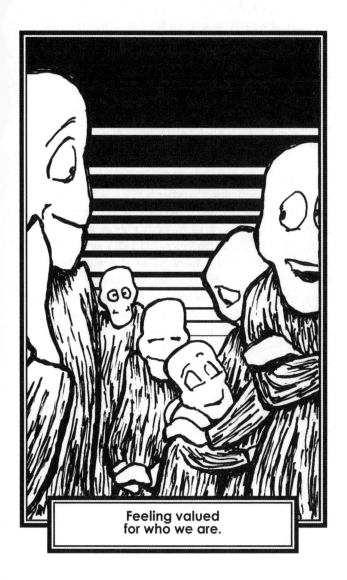

Feeling valued
for who we are.

collective has both been made possible by the emergence of the survivor movement and is a key foundation on which it is built. This is what is sometimes described as identity politics, where who we are and our associated experience is key to our political viewpoint, both shaping and unifying it. This tends to be defined in terms of political arguments and approaches which are based on self-identified social minority and social interest groups, usually associated with being marginalised or oppressed.

What mental health service users/survivors have in common is their experience and the resulting experiential knowledge born of direct experience. That is the basis of their movement. That shapes its focus and underpins its politics. This is the same as with other liberatory groupings such as the civil rights movement of black people, the feminist movement of women and the movement based on their sexuality of gay men, lesbians, bisexual and transgender people. All these groups of people have come together and acted politically together on the basis of who they are and the resulting oppression and discrimination that they have faced. The same is true of survivors and their movement. Psychiatric system survivor is both a personal and a political identity. They are unified by their experience of distress and of a psychiatric system and broader society both of which they experience as oppressive. Their politics are closely based on the personal as well as the political, unifying the two.

Chapter 7
From a medical to a social model

> Second, the social model refuses to see specific problems
> in isolation from the totality of disabling environments:
> hence the problem of unemployment does not just entail
> intervention in the social organisation of work and the
> operation of the labour market, but also in areas such as
> transport, education and culture.[1]
>
> *Mike Oliver*

The development of the mental health service user/survivor
movement has had many effects. As we have seen, it has
helped service users to gain a different, more confident and
positive understanding of themselves and their experience. It
has begun to influence practitioners and impact on policy
and practice. Its influence has grown to be international.
But perhaps the most important single result of the
development of the survivors' movement is that it makes it
possible to reframe mental health issues in new, different
and more helpful ways. It offers the prospect of at last
moving from a medical to a helpful social approach to
mental health issues. We have already touched more than
once on the medical model in relation to mental health
issues. This book has highlighted the dominance of the
medical model in the context of mental health and the
mental health system. What can't be overstated is the
pervasive and unhelpful nature of this model.

The negative nature of the medical model

In a two-year national study, service users/survivors and others were asked how they thought mental health issues were understood in society. The general consensus was that they were poorly understood and primarily associated with fear and danger. This appeared to originate from and be underpinned by a medicalised individual model of 'mental illness'. There was significant agreement that such a medicalised approach had few benefits to offer and was largely negative in effect.[2] Such a medical model was seen as all-pervasive in society. Professional approaches to mental health issues were also seen as being mainly medically based, seeing the problem as lying within the individual and responding primarily through the use of medication. Such professional interpretations were felt to have an important and unhelpful influence on public understandings. Among service users, the medical model was also seen as powerful; shaping, overshadowing and restricting their own understanding and attitudes. Without acknowledging the dominance of the medical model in mental health, it is difficult to explain or understand the current over-reliance in 'treatment' on drug 'therapies' or the predominating focus in mental health research on drug testing and its framing in terms of the diagnostic categories people are included in.

Participants in this study, in contrast, felt that a social approach to mental health issues brought with it a number of benefits. It was likely to lead to better understanding, better personal support, a service user focus in provision and could help change and improve wider attitudes by challenging narrow medicalised understandings of mental health. Service users felt that broader issues needed to be taken more account of to counter the individualisation of mental health issues. At the same time, there was a feeling among some mental health service users/survivors that it might be difficult for people to understand and implement a more social approach in a society strongly rooted in a medicalised individual model of mental illness.

A social model and mental health

There has long been some interest in and awareness of social issues in relation to mental health. But it has been marginalised by the medical model approaches.

The traditional social approach

At the same time, it may be argued that the emphasis here on the medical model in mental health overstates the issue; that there is a long and growing tradition of social approaches to and understandings of madness and distress, and that many psychiatrists and other clinicians are well aware of the role other broader issues can play in people's lives and experience beyond their personal difficulties. After all, there has been a distinct field of social psychiatry and some progressive psychiatrists and psychologists have shown interest in social approaches. There is no question that there has been an awareness of social issues in some mental health disciplines and professions for some time. But this has tended to focus on social issues as *factors* in the creation of mental health problems. It has tended still to take mental illness or disorder as a given – to accept the idea – rather than attempting to reconceptualise mental health within a social framework.

While mental health service users from this study and other discussions seem to be supportive of a more social understanding of mental health issues, discussion of such a social approach in mental health has so far been limited.

This is in sharp contrast to the disabled people's movement where such discussion has been central to its development. The social approach that they have developed has been ground-breaking in nature and implications.

The importance of the social model of disability

The social model of disability was developed by the disabled people's movement. It has had a major impact on public policy and understanding in the UK and internationally, leading to major new legislation, new policies, new support roles and new approaches to service provision. It challenged traditional Western understandings of disability. These focused on the individual, seeing disability as located within individual disabled people and resulting from some inherited or acquired disability which restricted what disabled people could do and could result in them being dependent and unable to live a 'normal' life. During the 20th century, such individualised understandings of disability were overlaid by the medicalised thinking of emerging medical professions which appropriated disability as an area of their expertise. The disabled people's movement saw this as resulting in a medicalised individual model of disability which conceived of disability as pathological and disabled people as requiring institutionalisation, rehabilitation and welfare support.[3,4,5]

The social model of disability which disabled activists developed instead drew a distinction between the physical, sensory or intellectual impairment or perceived impairment affecting an individual disabled person and the negative societal reaction to it. It is the latter which they conceived of as disability. Thus disability was understood as a discriminatory and oppressive response to people seen as having an impairment, rather than a characteristic attached to the individual. Discussion of the social model of disability among disability activists and in disability studies has been lively and fast-moving.[6] For disabled people, it has been a ground-breaking idea, shifting blame and responsibility for disability from the individual to the society and exploring the complex interrelations of the two. The social model of disability highlights the oppressive nature of the dominant social response to impairment, which excludes, segregates and stigmatises disabled people, creates barriers to their equality and participation and discriminates against them, restricting their human and civil rights. This approach to understanding has encouraged disabled people to highlight the problems they face as primarily a civil rights (rather than welfare) issue. There is no doubt that the social model of disability has influenced public understanding of disability, as well as many disabled people's own perceptions of themselves.

The social model of disability is a radical shift in understanding because it does not just take account of social factors while retaining an essentially medical approach to disability. It challenges such a medical approach because it takes account of the way that societal responses generate both understandings of disability and responses to it. It goes beyond the traditional 'nature versus nurture' approach to understanding people's situation as disabled people.

The social model of disability helps us to understand:

- the many barriers disabled people still face in society. These include social, economic, political and cultural barriers

- the discrimination that they face – the negative attitudes they encounter both from individuals and more broadly in society

- the oppressive way in which they can expect to be treated in society

- the way their human and civil rights tend to be restricted and undermined

All these barriers and issues, of course, can also be seen to be experienced by mental health service users/survivors, just as disabled people have highlighted the barriers restricting them. Most participants in the study referred to above felt that they experienced barriers as mental health service users.[7] Thus the social model of disability offers a helpful starting point and framework to develop in relation to the situation of mental health service users and madness and distress. It is easy to see how mental health service users are negatively affected by societal responses to them and the damaging effects these have. A social model of madness and distress is also likely to help us understand better:

- people's experience of madness and distress
- the societal barriers and discriminations operating in relation to madness and distress and their effects in disabling or 'maddening' people
- how some people's experience, perceptions and behaviour comes to be seen as 'mentally ill'
- why some groups (particularly black and minority ethnic people) face particular discrimination relating to madness and distress and the mental health system
- why madness and distress have also always been associated with and included people seen as non-conformist, resisting, disaffiliated and different

The development of such a social model of madness and distress also coincides with a broader and growing interest in social approaches to mental health. This has been signalled, for example, by the setting up of the Social Perspectives

Network to explore and develop more social approaches to mental health (http://www.spn.org.uk/) and the publication of new books on the subject.[8,9] While some survivor activists have been working to develop these ideas, as the national study showed, others less actively involved still seem to have concerns about such a model.[10] This reflects a similar situation with the initial development of the social model of disability, when many disabled people were wary or didn't understand it. Since then disabled people have increasingly described it as providing a 'light bulb' moment in their lives, offering a revelation which made it possible for them to challenge feelings of deficiency and blame and to think of themselves in new and positive ways. Far from being an abstract issue, it has a close bearing on people's ordinary day-to-day lives and understanding. The social model of disability does not seek to deny the individual experience of impairment and nor does a social model of madness and distress ignore the distress that people experience. Rather the aim is to challenge the oppression and discrimination both groups face as a result and to develop more appropriate responses to their circumstances and experiences.

Just as the social model of disability has demonstrated its revolutionary potential for disabled people's lives, so we can expect that a comparable social model of madness and distress could have the same potential for service users/survivors. It offers the basis for a completely different way of coming at mental health issues – one which prioritises service users' perspectives and puts them and their lives in a wider context. It points to different ways for people to understand themselves and each other and different ways of addressing their experience and circumstances. It is to this that we turn next.

Chapter 8
Developing a new vision: Principles for the future

> My hope is for people to say, 'Do you know, 50 years
> ago, we used to say to people who'd been traumatised
> and abused and had terrible emotional problems, we used
> to say, "You're a schizophrenic or a manic depressive and
> you'll always be like that".' We will look back and be
> horrified at the kind of things we do to one another today.[1]
> *Survivor*

The focus in 'mental health' has often seemed backward-looking. Much energy, from both reformers and service users/survivors themselves, has been put into trying to improve the psychiatric system. Of course there have been some improvements. Some service users/survivors have accessed forms of support, particularly 'talking therapies', which were not previously available to them. Some new drugs have been developed which, used sensitively, have improved the lives of some service users/survivors. There isn't quite the sense there once was that people who get caught up in the system are irretrievably lost to it.

However, it is difficult to feel that progress has matched that in other areas of medicine with which psychiatry might reasonably be compared. More often it feels like two steps forward and another step back, with constant cuts and changes, reductions in services, a constant need for 'through-put' – for people to move on – and less time with support workers. As has been said, the psychiatric system seems to have an amazing capacity to resist progressive reform.

But, as we have seen, there is now a chance to start from a radically different paradigm. Service users/survivors and their organisations have developed their own ideas and values; their own theories and analysis; their own services and forms of support; their own arts and culture; their own forms of research and evaluation; their own literature and materials. In a relatively short time, they have challenged old assumptions, pioneered new approaches and impacted on policy and practice. But they have faced many obstacles and difficulties in taking forward their own proposals.

Their own innovative ideas and developments provide a basis for a new service user-led social paradigm, based on a social approach to 'mental health' or, as many survivors prefer to call it, madness and distress. A range of elements for such an approach can now be identified from existing experience. Most if not all of these elements already have a track record of development. However, what hasn't yet happened is for them to be put together as part of a properly supported strategic approach to 'mental health' policy and practice development and reform. They have yet to become central in mental health policy and practice so that they can be an everyday routine reality and choice for *everyone* who may come the way of the mental health system – as both service provider and service user. The ideas and developments set out here build on the experience of many service users, as well as of innovative policy makers, practitioners and managers. The values, principles and proposals offered here have been the subject of many people's thinking and many formal debates and informal discussions.

In this third part of the book, we look at what policy and provision in relation to madness and distress might look like if they were built on the understanding, knowledge and experience which is now available, particularly the emerging and developing ideas of service users, instead of being limited by our inheritance from the past. We begin with the kind of principles and values that such a new approach to madness and distress might be based upon.

The principles or values of such a socially based system are likely to include:

- prioritising self-advocacy
- being rights-based
- building on the philosophy of independent living
- self-management and self-support
- commitment to anti-oppressive practice
- supporting race equality and cultural diversity
- minimising compulsion
- breaking the bad/mad link
- prioritising participation
- equalising power relations

We now look in more detail at each of these in turn.

Prioritising self-advocacy

At the heart of every movement, and this is as true for survivors as any other group struggling against oppression and discrimination, is the need to be able to speak and act for yourself rather than having others speak for you. This is a fundamental starting point for regaining control of your life. It is a core principle for service user/survivor-led rather than service system-led ideas and understandings for making sense of madness and distress and changing the situation of mental health service users/survivors. This development has widely come to be called self-advocacy.

Advocacy more generally is essential in any system which seeks to safeguard service users' rights and which can impose restrictions on these rights. With the extension of compulsory treatment into the community and the rising number of service users/survivors who are becoming subject to sections (compulsory treatment under the Mental Health Act), the need for advocacy has become increasingly important. It was meant to be provided alongside the extension of compulsory 'treatment' but this has not been adequately developed. Advocacy, to be effective, needs to:

- be independent (of the service system)

- be of good quality – employing skilled, trained and qualified advocates. There need to be recognised qualifications for advocates to ensure the provision of a high quality and reliable service.

- be available both on demand and without request. Not everyone knows about advocacy or the benefits it can offer. It is important that it is offered routinely and that while it may of course be refused, it is always available. Without such independent advocacy, there can be no assumption that service users have been able to give their informed consent.

- be ongoing and available prior to a problem or a crisis. Advocacy is often only available when something has gone seriously wrong or people's rights are being removed. All the evidence indicates that good advocacy is based upon the quality of relationship between advocate and service user. It is essential that people can have access to an advocate prior to problems emerging.

• values service users' direct experience. Many service users particularly value advocacy provided by people with shared understandings and experience. Advocacy policy should take this into account and support and encourage the recruitment and training of suitable candidates with experience as service users.

• be provided on an equal basis for black and minority ethnic service users. There is a serious lack of black and minority ethnic advocates for and provided by black and minority ethnic service users. Black and ethnic minority service users often value having black and minority ethnic advocates and advocacy services and this option needs to be readily available.

There are two other key requirements for good advocacy. First, advocacy should never be seen as an alternative to making services and processes as accessible, empowering and user friendly as possible, so that as far as possible any service user can negotiate them on his/her own. Second, and this is key, all forms of advocacy (legal, professional, peer and citizen advocacy) should primarily be directed to supporting self-advocacy; that is to say, the capacity of each individual service user to speak and act on their own behalf.

Being rights-based

Traditionally, responses to welfare service users like mental health service users/survivors and disabled people were based on definitions of their needs by outside 'experts'. First disabled people and then other groups felt that this created many problems and instead developed a rights-based approach, taking as the key yardstick for policy and practice how far it secured or undermined their civil and human rights. This included rights like:

- the right to freedom of movement
- the right to life
- the right to sexuality and reproduction
- freedom from want
- freedom from discrimination and to have effective redress against it
- to vote and participate in the political process
- the support that is needed to live your life on equal terms
- freedom of choice and opportunities
- the right to work
- freedom of information

This is why the disabled people's movement campaigned for civil rights and freedom of information legislation. In the UK, reflecting international developments, such aspirations have now been taken forward to some extent by the extended provisions of the Disability Discrimination legislation and the Disability Equality Duty, as well as the Human Rights Act.

Many mental health service users/survivors are categorised as disabled people and have entitlements under the Human Rights and Disability Discrimination Acts to disability benefits and to the direct payments and personal budget schemes pioneered by disabled people, which enable service users to shape their own package of support and, with the assistance they need, to control it themselves. A rights-based approach to mental health policy and practice highlights the importance of evaluating policy and provision in terms of the degree to which they support (or obstruct) service users' full and equal citizenship in society.

The philosophy of independent living

The idea of independent living is a simple but revolutionary one. It is a philosophy that was originally inspired by the disabled people's movement. It also works helpfully for people who use mental health services. It follows from the social model of disability. It is based on a belief that disabled people should be enabled to live their lives on as equal terms as possible alongside non-disabled people. It doesn't say how you should live or that you should live the same as anyone else. Instead it says you should have the same choice as anyone who isn't disabled (or here, who isn't a mental health service user), as far as possible. The philosophy of independent living turns traditional notions of independence on their head. It is not preoccupied with the individual, or narrow ideas of personal autonomy. It does not mean 'standing on your own two feet or managing on your own'. Instead of seeing the service user as having a defect or deficiency requiring care, it highlights the need to ensure that they have the support they need to live their lives as fully as possible, on equal terms and interdependently with others.[2] This support is not expected to come from required to be unpaid family members or 'informal carers'.

The philosophy rejects the concept of care and replaces it with the idea of support. It sees independence as meaning being in a position to make your own decisions, rather than having to do everything for yourself.[3,4] Instead of people being assessed on the basis of what they aren't able to do in order to qualify for 'care', under this model, support is provided to enable them to live their lives as fully as possible, as they wish to. There are two inter-related and key aspects to the philosophy of independent living. These are:

- ensuring people the support that they need under their control to be able to live their lives as fully as they can, on as equal terms as possible, with non-disabled people

- equalising their access to mainstream policy, services and amenities, like housing, health, education, employment and recreation

This emphasises the relevance of independent living as a value base across public policy, as well as specifically in relation to human services. In England, a governmental Independent Living Strategy with cross-departmental support signed up to these values,[5] although again it needs to be said that public services are still a long way from being organised and provided on a basis consistent with this.

You can see how this will also apply to people experiencing madness and distress. The aim should be to try and ensure that they can have the support they need to live as full and good a life as they can. It recognises that they may still face difficulties from their experience of distress, but is based on trying to make sure that these can be minimised as far as possible and that lack of support is not made an additional problem for people.

Recovery
Independent living is not the only big 'new' idea which has developed and which has relevance to mental health issues and service users/survivors. Another is 'recovery'. This reflects the desire of service users and their movements to be recognised as active, contributing citizens. It has gained some support from service users. But it has mainly been shaped and advanced by state and service providers, rather than service users and their organisations and can be seen to

be at least ambiguous and contentious in its role and purpose.

The idea of recovery has recently gained major interest in UK mental health policy and practice. There is talk of a 'recovery movement'.[6] Many service users value the idea of recovery because it does not write them off as irreparably damaged or defective, but instead offers hope and the possibility of positive outcomes for their lives.[7] Other survivors, however, are highly critical of the concept's essentially medicalised basis and the associated emphasis on 're-ablement' and moving people to employment. While the philosophy of independent living developed by disabled people emphasises people's potentially continuing need for support to live their lives to the full, recovery instead implies that such support may become unnecessary and be withdrawn as people 'recover'. For this reason, some survivors see recovery as at least consistent with and in some cases supportive of the reactionary agenda of cuts, integration into the labour market and increasing reliance on people's self-help and 'looking after themselves'.

Self-management and self-support

Service users have a central role to play in 'shaping their own lives'. Self-support and self-management has often been taken to mean a kind of 'self-help' approach, where the service user 'graduates' from formal support and manages on their own. This is often a bridge too far for service users and their loved ones and is actually experienced as withdrawal and being left to try and cope and manage on their own.

There are more positive meanings for self-management and self-support that need to be developed instead. These are not concerned with trying to manage on your own, but of being in control, as far as possible and desired, with the support you need, to manage your own life. Living as full and secure a life as possible on a sustainable basis can often also mean having support available at those times when you might again need it. This can be both formal and informal support. Just knowing the support can be available is sometimes enough in itself. The forms such support can take may include:

1. developing skills to maintain and run your own life

2. playing the pivotal role (with support as needed) to run and negotiate the range of service interventions that might be needed in your life. The service user becomes the ringmaster rather than the passive bystander of what is happening in their life; having a shaping role in:

   - the nature and kind of support they receive
   - any medication they receive
   - the workers who work with them
   - the particular service providers they access

The service user is no longer the fly in the spider's web of services. Instead he or she can become the spider developing their own web of support and assistance, consistent with their own definitions of what they want and need. As has been said, to do this, they may also need capacity building or ongoing support in the form of advocacy, advice and information.

A recent emphasis in health and social care policy discussions on 'personalisation' and 'personal budgets' chimes with ideas of self-management and self-support. The idea is that services should be shaped by and 'customised' to what each person needs, rather than people being fitted into a 'service-led' system. A key method for realising such personalisation has been seen as personal budgets, which offer people who are eligible a sum of money to spend on whatever support they would find most helpful. We look at this development in more detail in the next chapter.

Based on anti-oppressive practice

As we saw earlier, mental health policy and practice continue to be beset with problems of inequality and discrimination. The particular problems facing black people and minority ethnic groups in the mental health system, as well as the particular difficulties facing women, particularly as mothers and in relation to safety, are well documented. A systematic approach in mental health practice to challenging discrimination based on difference on grounds of 'race', gender, sexuality, age, class, culture, faith, belief and disability is required. Such an approach has been developed in the fields of social work and social care practice. It will need to extend across occupational and professional groups and at all levels in the mental health system. It will need to be supported at organisational as well as individual levels.

Anti-oppressive practice needs to be linked with a systematic process of ongoing monitoring, evaluation, review and reward. Anti-oppressive practice does not generally sit comfortably with the restriction of people's rights, so the two concerns need to be considered in relation to each other. Service users and their organisations, rather than professionals, need to play a central role in shaping and developing anti-oppressive practice to ensure it meets their rights and needs.[8]

Supporting race equality and cultural diversity

The mental health system has so far demonstrated a frequent failure to address issues of cultural diversity and race equality successfully. There can be little doubt that it is a system that continues to be overshadowed by institutionalised racism. Black and minority ethnic service users (particularly some groups, like African-Caribbean young men and Irish people) have particularly negative experiences of the mental health system. Black service users face disproportionately high risks of death in the system: of being restricted to chemical 'treatments' and of over-prescription. While there is now a large and growing number of black and minority ethnic practitioners, including psychiatrists and other professionals, psychiatry continues to be essentially Eurocentric in its orientation and operation.

Addressing issues of race equality and cultural diversity must be a priority for any new approach to mental health policy and practice. While there have been numerous government initiatives along these lines, so far they have not been successful. This commitment needs to be built into new social approaches to madness and distress. Black and minority ethnic service users and their organisations must be fully and effectively involved in efforts to reform the mental health system and to achieve the required commitment to race equality in its process, operation, capacity and goals.

In their definitive study of the survivor movement, Jan Wallcraft and her colleagues highlighted both the discriminatory nature of the psychiatric system and how much more work is still needed for the survivor movement to be fully inclusive and proactive in addressing diversity. This includes tackling barriers and discriminations that operate in relation to all the equality issues including, of course, gender and sexuality issues as well as those of race equality.[9]

Minimising compulsion

Historically, almost invariably systems set up in response to madness and subsequently 'mental illness' have included strong elements of compulsion. Sometimes these have overshadowed and shaped the whole system, giving rise to the segregated and regulatory 'asylum' institutions established in the 19th century, where the overall regime was conditioned by concerns to secure, separate, morally educate, discipline and sometimes punish inmates. The concern of systems for the 'mad' and 'insane' to maintain social control has often spilled over into the imposition of punitive and abusive regimes. Such abusive regimes can be identified from the 15th century to the present.

Compulsion and the restriction of service users' rights continue to be aspects of current mental health systems of increasing importance. In England, forensic services and restrictions on people's rights have grown in scale rather than diminished with any assumed improvement in understanding and therapy. This has been underpinned and reinforced by current concerns about the risk posed by mental health service users. In the present political and media climate, there seems little likelihood of compulsion ending in the psychiatric system. The immediate goal, however, must be to question and minimise it. The longer-term goal should be to end it. There are other ways of ensuring that people do not harm themselves or others than through the practice of forcible or compulsory 'treatment'. The concept is a contradiction in terms. Alternatives include:

- providing rapid, appropriate and adequate support in response to people's requests to prevent them reaching crisis

- routine and effective use (and adherence to requests set out in) to crisis cards and advance directives

- the use of the provisions of the criminal justice system where people break the law and/or pose a threat to others

- ensuring the availability of valued and safe crisis, emergency and other provision for service users encountering serious difficulties

Where service users' rights continue to be restricted, such provisions need to be accompanied by adequate safeguards which ensure:

- immediate independent advocacy and support
- rapid processes of hearing and review
- rights to appeal and independent representation

Breaking the bad/mad link

Since the policy shift from large institutions to 'care in the community', mental health service users have increasingly been associated, by politicians and the right-wing media, with violence, homicide, risk and threat to 'public safety'. While there is no evidence of any increase in violence or homicide from service users, this association has increasingly shaped policy responses and media presentations of mental health issues. It led to proposals for new legislation which generated unprecedented concerns about increased restrictions on the rights of mental health service users and widespread fears that many more service users will be drawn into the net of compulsion. Such legislation was then introduced and at least some of these fears have been justified. The lesson of numerous inquiries has been that homicides by mental health service users have tended to be linked with the failure of services to provide help when sought.

The assumed link between mental health service users and dangerousness has re-emerged to shape and dominate mental health policy practice and thinking. It creates a damaging prospect for the many thousands of service users who pose no threat to anyone. It is likely to increase the stigma faced by service users and make many reluctant to seek support from the mental health system.

However there are more fundamental issues here which need to be re-examined. First, it is hardly surprising if service users are associated with 'pathological' and deviant behaviour, when their conceptualisation is based on a model of 'mental illness' which assumes pathology. Second, violence has increasingly been medicalised in Western societies like the UK, on the basis of unevidenced assumptions that 'you must be mad to be so bad'. The medical model of mental illness is increasingly associated with violence. Thus, for example:

- common (physiological and psychological) responses to extreme threat and danger are reconceived as a form of mental disorder: 'post-traumatic stress disorder'

- 'mental disorder' is offered without reliable or consistent independent criteria or evidence to support it as an explanation for violence

- 'mental illness' and 'mental disorder' are routinely introduced as legal defences for criminal and violent behaviour

- committing violent acts without remorse is identified as a form of 'severe and dangerous personality disorder'

- being subjected to sexual and other violent abuse or assault (especially in childhood) is offered as a sufficient predictor or explanation for an individual's own subsequent abusive or violent behaviour

- the perpetration of child sexual abuse is identified as a category of 'mental disorder'

This requires fundamental reviews of:

- the concept of 'personality disorder' and 'borderline personality disorder'

- routine tendencies to associate 'mental illness' with violence, without reliable independent evidence

- the common use of 'mental disorder' as a defence for violent and sexual attacks and abuse

Prioritising participation

User involvement, empowerment and partnership have all become 'buzz words' in mental health. Yet still in wider society, mental health service users face some of the most serious problems of exclusion, stigma and powerlessness. While efforts have been made to increase the involvement of service users in mental health services, their position and status in society are still largely marginal.

Prioritising the participation of mental health service users/survivors offers an effective basis for challenging this situation. Instead of seeing participation as merely an add-on component to service provision, it needs to become a central concern for policy in the widest sense. Existing government requirements for the participation and partnership of mental health service users can provide an effective lever to achieve this. Participation needs to be recognised as both a central concern in the process and as a key purpose of policy, provision and practice. In this way, participation can provide a central means by which service users can:

- exert influence over their experience of and negotiations with the mental health system

- influence decision-making processes in the mental health system and other policies and services impacting on their lives

It should also be developed as a priority goal, to ensure that mental health service users:

- have the greatest possible opportunities to participate fully in all aspects of society according to their wishes and abilities, for example, in education, employment, recreation, in networks, social and family life and in their communities

In Chapter 10, we discuss 'user-controlled organisations'. These offer a key route to effective participation in every sense.

Equalising power relations

Experience of madness and distress is often, but not always, a disempowering experience. Frequently, however, experience of the mental health system adds to rather than reduces this sense of powerlessness. As we have seen, it becomes another problem to be dealt with, rather than feeling like part of a solution. If mental health services are to support people's well-being and act as a positive rather than negative experience, a help rather than a burden, then they need to be a positive in people's lives. If they are to achieve that, then they will need to be based on a fundamental commitment to equalise relationships within them. This can be seen as a key problem in existing services, which helps to explain the frequent problems of abuse, violence and poor conditions that service users report. Mental health services have frequently tended to be institutionalised and all the evidence is that such institutionalised services have the most difficulty ensuring and maintaining equal power relationships. The tendency within existing services may be to inequality because of existing inequality of power, status and credibility between service users, providers and professionals, but these can be challenged. Their operation must be regularly and routinely audited at all levels to establish how much this happens and to stop it continuing.

There are also other ways of ensuring that people can work in more equal and collaborative ways, which have been developed in other fields and where there have also been some pioneering initiatives in mental health provision. These include:

- increasing the involvement of people with experience as service users as trainers and educators in professional and occupational training and education

- encouraging the recruitment of people with service-user experience and appropriate skills to the mental health workforce

- rewarding workers for working in more participatory and inclusive ways as part of qualification requirements, performance review and promotion processes

• developing de-institutionalised approaches to support and services which provide 'open' rather than closed regimes, encouraging services, service workers and users to be in more routine contact with the wider world

All of these will build understanding and challenge disempowering barriers between mental health services and those they are intended to support.

Chapter 9
Developing a new vision: Survivor-led approaches to support

> Patient-controlled services: A real alternative to the institutions that destroy the confident independence of so many.[1]
> *Judi Chamberlin*

In the last chapter we looked at the kind of principles and values that follow from a survivor-led and social approach to madness and distress. We now consider the sort of support and provision that the evidence from and experience of service users/survivors and their organisations suggests is likely to be helpful for the future as the basis for improving the control they have over their lives and the quality of their support. If the old system has often seemed preoccupied with controlling and individualising people, then as Judi Chamberlin said, for the future, 'liberation is the goal' and it is most likely to be achieved through our own efforts as mental health service users/survivors.[2]

The elements that will go to make up the practice and provision of such an alternative approach to madness and distress are likely to include:

- being based on self-defined needs
- user-controlled and self-run services
- peer support

- valuing holistic and complementary approaches
- user-led training and education
- self-run schemes for personal support
- encouraging community development approaches
- the development of new roles and new approaches

All of these are about ensuring people the kind of support that they need to live their lives as well as they can and to be in a position to make informed judgements and decisions about what will most help. Taken together they make it possible for as many people as possible to be included in and benefit from such a new holistic approach to support. At the heart of them all lies the idea and achievement of user-controlled or self-run services, so particular attention is paid to these here. But the story starts with people being given the chance to work out what they want and what would most help them.

Being based on self-defined needs

At present, people mainly go to services and services offer what they are used to providing or what they think service users need. We know that this doesn't work well. But equally, just being told that you can make choices and have what you want doesn't necessarily mean much if you have low expectations, little idea or information about what might be possible and have spent years in disempowering and institutionalising situations. People need first to be in a position to make meaningful choices.

People's human and civil rights, and safeguarding them, need to be central in a reformed approach to mental health. The mental health system has traditionally been based on ideas of 'need'. This approach has tended to have a number of shortcomings. It has generally been based on the definitions and judgements of professionals and organisations employing a medical model. This approach has emphasised people's inabilities and deficiencies, rather than their capacity. In order to qualify for support, people have had to demonstrate their deficiencies. This has worked against preventive approaches to madness and distress. It frequently means that people cannot access a small amount of support to enable them to maintain their lives and activities, which then puts these in jeopardy.

As Judi Chamberlin said many years back now, 'The definition of need would come from the client'.[3] It is important to move to a model based on self-definition of needs where, with appropriate advocacy, information and support, service users are able to identify what support they would want to do the things they would like to do. This was the aspiration at the heart of the care management and care programme approach introduced in 1993 with the Community Care reforms.

To work this will need:

- independent, reliable and accessible information
- independent advocacy, including peer advocacy and support for self-advocacy
- independent (non-medicalised) assessment

Disabled people's organisations have begun to develop roles, training and accreditation enabling service users to provide such support on an independent basis, informed by shared experience. In this way service users who need and want support are much more likely to be at the starting line knowing what they want and confident enough to be assertive in getting it.

User-controlled and self-run services

At the heart of a radically altered support for people with madness and distress and experience of the psychiatric system are self-run or user-controlled services. They are absolutely key to transforming mental health policy and practice and the lives of mental health service users/survivors.

There is now a long track record of mental health service users/survivors pioneering their own user-controlled services. The famous American survivor, Judi Chamberlin, was writing about 'patient-controlled services' in her groundbreaking book, *On Our Own*, first published in 1978.[4] This can be seen as part of a broader development of user-controlled services developed by service users and disabled people. This has a history of more than 20 years' innovation. These include safe houses and crisis houses, drop-in and day centres, help lines, advocacy and peer-support schemes, residential, housing and employment projects, environmental and gardening schemes.

In the mental health field, user-controlled services have tended to break out of the narrow medicalised approach to responding to mental health problems, instead framing support in broader social terms that address the wider problems and barriers that service users highlight. They have been organised as cooperatives, social enterprise schemes and charitable organisations. They can be, as Judi Chamberlin highlighted, a network of provision and support, flexible so that people can move within it as they need more or less or different kinds of support.[5] Such services have been run and managed by service users with service user workers. We also have reliable evidence about such user-controlled services. A major national study supported by the Big Lottery was carried out which explored the views of all stakeholders involved with such

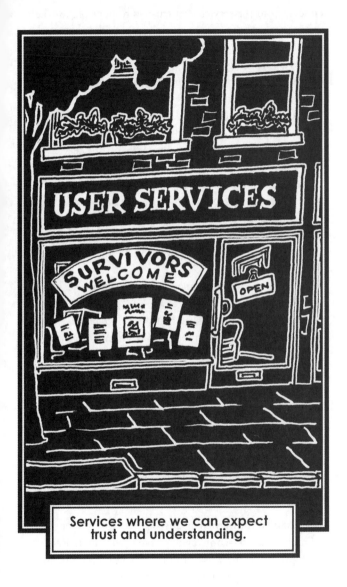

Services where we can expect
trust and understanding.

services, from the service user trustees responsible for their governance and the user practitioners providing them, to, crucially, the service users who accessed them. The results were overwhelmingly positive. Service users valued such services, felt that they were more supportive and sensitive than other traditional arrangements and highlighted their benefits. Such services were particularly popular among service users and improved their quality of life. This has important economic and social benefits for the service user, their family and the local community.[6]

Judi Chamberlin's inspiring work is still invaluable for understanding the ground-breaking role of user-controlled services. She based it on the US experience while also looking at developments in other countries. Her experience connects closely with that in the UK. As she wrote:

> Patient-controlled alternatives can provide services to people without the demoralising consequences of the authoritarian, hierarchical structures of traditional mental health services. When the emphasis is on people helping one another, the gulf between 'patient' and 'staff' disappears. Someone can seek help from others without being thought of as sick or helpless.[7]

> Non-professional, client-controlled services don't divide people into 'sick' and 'well', 'helper' and 'helped'. They see every person as having a combination of strengths and weaknesses, and the need for help in one area does not negate the ability to help others also.[8]

Judi Chamberlin warned against services that presented themselves as 'user-controlled' where service users were employed to do the work or did it as volunteers, but control stayed with traditional mental health professionals.

She was suspicious of 'alternative' services based on 'partnership' or collaboration models with professionals, believing that the latter tended always to take over. She argued instead for a separatist model where 'ex-patients provide support for one another and run the service ... they provide a real alternative to the dehumanising effects of mental health 'care'.[9]

> On the other hand, the alternatives built on the supportive and separatist models – the true alternatives – have been designed by ex-patients who are not merely passive recipients of a service but who are actively involved in running it ... In the professional versions of alternatives ... the professional is always the senior partner.[10]

Tina Coldham, Chair of the National Survivor User Network and long-term activist, makes similar points from a UK perspective:

> To some, user-led services might seem like the lunatics running the asylum. However, mad people are moved to provide user-led provision for their peers for very good reasons. Firstly, we can have enormous insight into our distress and develop incredible empathy towards others as a result of this. Secondly, because we are grounded in our experiences, users can be very objective and committed to making what matters work. More so, we harbour a deeper understanding of what matters and therefore are driven by a passion for getting it right, particularly when we feel others miss the point. User involvement is a means to an end; that end is people being able to get on with their lives mentally well. However, involvement often becomes a whole industry with a purpose of its own, and doesn't actually impact upon people's lives as the end product.

Users and survivors are brave to challenge the vast mental
health system from within. Some of us are running
alternatives to this as a way of challenging the status quo
in a positive manner that can have real impact upon
people's lives. We can be 'madly' creative and innovative
in developing solutions to our problems, and in doing so,
inspire others, and develop user leadership. I was once
told 'If you want commitment, get people who have been
committed!' What more can I say?

Service users and their organisations have found it very
difficult to get the funding and other support to develop
their own services on any scale. Their status has often been
precarious and valued services have closed through failure to
secure their funding. Service users are thus frequently
denied this choice and even where such services are
available, mainstream services are sometimes unaware of
their existence and don't refer service users to them.

Over a number of years now, successive UK
governments have argued the importance of services being
available from a wide range of providers. They have
highlighted the problems they associate with the state
dominating the provision of services. They have frequently
called for an expanded role for the voluntary sector. There
has been a massive expansion in private sector provision,
which has become the major provider of social care services.
This pressure for a move away from state provision is closely
in tune with the development of service user-controlled
services. Yet the irony is that over this period, such services
still remain marginal, both in mental health and wider
health and social care provision. This is not for want of
service users trying. Service users and their organisations
have worked hard to expand the kind of non-medicalised
provision that they have shown a particular capacity to

provide successfully. However, they have continued to face big barriers. As Colin Barnes of the Centre for Disability Studies at Leeds University says of the pioneering developments by disabled people:

> In spite of entrenched opposition from established service providers, services such as Disability Information and Advice Lines (DIAL), peer counselling and support facilities, integrated accessible housing schemes for disabled and non-disabled people, direct payment schemes for personal assistance and technical aids and equipment, were all pioneered and provided by grass roots CIL-type [Centres for Independent Living] groups during the 1970s and 80s.

User-controlled services have received little support or encouragement in local or national commissioning policies, for all their rhetoric of challenging traditional patterns of service provision and the 'monopoly' of state provision. The typical pattern of provision is still based on large for-profit organisations and traditional charities, purchased through block commissioning for economies of scale, standardised for large numbers of people. This advantages the lowest bidders who tend to employ workers at the lowest rates and with the poorest conditions.

The same obstacles in the way of user-controlled services that Judi Chamberlin identified more than 30 years ago still apply. It is difficult to secure funding, professionals are often opposed and service users may be lacking in confidence and capacity. While there have been outstanding examples of innovation from user-controlled services, these have tended to be insecure and have often been short-lived for want of wider official support. The insecurity and under-funding of such services means that their skilled and experienced user workers often have to move on to conventional services, to ensure some job security in their own lives. Often the aspirations to provide truly user-controlled services have been subverted because service users haven't been granted the status or credibility to take them forward and more traditional organisations have taken over such initiatives and ideas, undermining their user-controlled principles in the process.

There are likely to be growing opportunities for user-controlled services through the expansion of personal budgets and self-directed support schemes which we discuss in more detail in this chapter. They offer people the chance to choose their own 'package of support' and we can expect many people to opt for user-controlled support. Whether governments will support this wholeheartedly is another matter and so here is a further issue where service users/survivors can make a difference by making their voices heard loud and clear.

A strategic approach to supporting the development of user-controlled and self-run services is key for the future. This will need the allocation of specific (secure) funding to kick-start such provision. Such services also offer important employment, training and career opportunities for mental health service users/survivors. More support and evaluation will be needed to maximise these opportunities and to enhance skill development and career opportunities for service users. They offer a ground-breaking and unique way in which 'the helped' can be helpers and the helping helped.

Peer support

There are many approaches to peer support. These can be more and less formal. Service users/survivors have long highlighted the value they get from the support that they can offer each other because of the shared understandings and experience, which provide a key basis for trust-building and mutuality. Some service users develop 'mentoring' relationships with others, which provide guidance and support. Others have formed counselling relationships with each other based on friendship and shared experience. For example, a long-term mental health service user described to me an arrangement that he and a couple of survivors had used over several years. Initially it was a support group where they would meet and then it became a virtual support group where they did not physically meet. They would begin by taking turns talking about their situation without interruption for about five minutes, only occasionally giving feedback to each other. People were listened to and found it really helpful to talk about what was happening to them in an atmosphere of non-judgement and understanding.

It is also worth quoting Anne Wilson (the pseudonym of a mental health service user/survivor) at length about the positives she has gained from 'co-counselling':

> I was a mental health service user and was well and truly caught up in the psychiatric system. I met someone who was involved in co-counselling and was really interested in what she told me. When I told the mental health professionals working with me that I wanted to try co-counselling, all of them advised against it because they said people like me (with 'schizophrenia') 'needed trained mental health professionals, not amateurs'.
>
> Seven years later, I picked up the phone and dialled the number in an advert for a CCI (Co-Counselling International) 'fundamentals' course. The person who answered the phone wasn't at all fazed by my saying that I'd had psychiatric treatment in the past (I had by then taken myself off medication and because I'd moved around

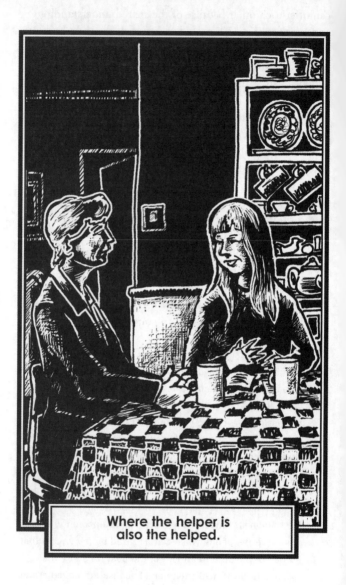

Where the helper is
also the helped.

the country several times the mental health professionals had lost track of me). She did say that in order to do co-counselling, I would need to have the emotional resources to listen to and support another person, which I felt I did, so I joined the course.

Doing co-counselling fundamentals training has to be the best thing I have ever done in my life, but probably not for the reason you think!

Co-counsellors work in pairs and halfway through, 'client' and 'counsellor' swap places so you each spend an equal amount of time as both client and counsellor. It is therefore a relationship of equals and there is no possibility of an 'expert' or 'professional' telling you what is 'wrong with you', as when it is your turn to be the client, you are in charge. This was a revelation, but nothing like as much of a revelation as the most important thing for me about co-counselling which was hearing other people talk about their experiences and concerns when they were the client and I was the counsellor. What I realised was that a lot of the 'symptoms' and strange perceptions I experienced (which psychiatrists had attributed to 'schizophrenia' in my case) were in fact quite common experiences – I realised this because I co-counselled with many, many people who during the course of their co-counselling sessions spoke about being in stressful situations and experiencing some of what I experienced, maybe in not such an extreme way or over such extended periods, but nevertheless very similar experiences to my own. I can't tell you what they said as the content of co-counselling sessions is strictly confidential, and confidentiality is something which co-counsellors take very seriously.

Through co-counselling therefore I came to see myself as a 'normal' person. This was a fantastic achievement given all the negative and damning roles I'd been assigned by the psychiatrists; roles which I had also deeply internalised. And I also made many friends.

That's not to say however that co-counselling has been a bed of roses, for (just as in the population at large) there are some co-counsellors who hold 'mentalist' attitudes. For me, the best co-counsellors have been people who have also had encounters with psychiatry themselves. Being involved in CCI [Co-Counselling International – http://www.co-counselling.org.uk] has also enabled me to develop friendship networks locally, nationally and internationally.

Valuing holistic and complementary approaches

The medical base of mental health policy and thinking – the tendency to separate the mind from the body – has encouraged the prevailing medicalised 'treatment' responses to people included as mental health service users. This has been reinforced by the bureaucratic tendency to organise and compartmentalise according to policy and administrative concerns, rather than on the basis of individual lives, rights, wants and needs.

When the government made an attempt to move away from the dominance of drug therapy to introduce more 'talking therapies', it seemed to do this in a similarly mechanistic way. The Improving Access to Psychological Therapies programme (IAPT) placed a strong emphasis on cognitive behavioural therapy (CBT) rather than the wider range of such therapies, offered a very limited number of sessions and used practitioners who tended to have a narrow range of skills and experience. Service users/survivors voiced concerns that these sessions raised issues for them without further support being available for them to deal with these issues.

Traditional 'scientific' prejudices also discouraged the development and application of the wide range of complementary therapies available. They have also come in for criticism because they often do not show well in typical randomised control trial approaches to evaluation. Although such approaches to support are still treated with suspicion in the mainstream, this has begun to change. User-controlled and voluntary organisations as well as private practitioners are increasingly offering such approaches. They are also entering mainstream statutory services. But they are far from being a routine option for many service users, especially not for the majority on low income. Such services are particularly suited and receptive to an holistic approach to emotional and mental distress. Policy and provision needs to develop a more holistic approach to the rights and needs of service users. This includes:

- seeing the individual as a person, not a collection of problems, symptoms or deficits.

- integrating policies; recognising the interrelation of different aspects of the person's life and connecting policies to fit these. It is not enough to see policy and provision for mental health service users as the sole concern of the National Health Service or social care. The wide range of relevant policy areas, including income maintenance, public transport, leisure and recreation, education and employment, must also be taken into account and audited against the inclusive and participatory goals of such an alternative mental health system.

- giving equal recognition to complementary approaches to healing valued by service users, enabling them to be evaluated in appropriate ways.

User-led training and education

Service users, their organisations, progressive practitioners and service organisations have long argued that involving service users in staff and professional education and training can play a crucial role in improving service cultures and making them more 'user-centred'. Even on a piecemeal basis, the introduction of 'user training', the development of a growing number of user trainers and the development of 'training for user trainers' have all made a valuable impact on mental health provision and practice. What is still needed is a coherent and systematic approach to user involvement in mental health training which goes far beyond bringing in service users to offer one-off sessions on their personal experience.

The new three-year social work qualification introduced in 2003 requires service user involvement in *all* aspects of professional education and it is such a coherent approach which is needed across mental health occupations, professions and disciplines. It is greatly valued by students on such social work courses. This type of approach needs to include user involvement in recruitment, curriculum development, teaching, assessment and accreditation. It should draw on materials produced by mental health service users and their organisations to complement other sources of learning material. Such materials are now increasingly being produced.

Self-run schemes for personal support

The main way in which the disabled people's movement in the UK has been able to advance the idea of 'independent living' based on a social model of disability has been through the introduction of 'direct payments' or 'self-run personal assistance' schemes. What these mean essentially is that the individual service user, after assessment, receives an allocation of state funding directly, with which they are then able to purchase the 'package of support' which *they* want, to meet their support needs as they define them. Disabled people have often used this money to employ 'personal assistants' (who they hire and fire) to meet their support requirements. So far, such direct payments schemes, which have subsequently been extended by legislation to become a mandatory option for a wider range of service users including many mental health service users, have represented the strongest expression of 'user-controlled' support for health and social care service users.

More recently, much more emphasis has been placed on such schemes by policymakers and politicians under the heading of personal and individual budgets and 'self-directed support' schemes. They are now available both through social care and health services. They can provide marvellous opportunities for mental health service users to get the kind of socially based support that the traditional mental health system has so often failed to provide. However, there are still several major obstacles in the way of this happening. First, the level of funding provided is now more likely to be based on what limited money is available, rather than what support people actually need to live their lives to the best. Second, restrictions are often placed on what kind of support service users are allowed to purchase because of assumptions either that they are not sufficiently responsible or that there might be a media backlash to the kind of support services they find helpful.

As yet, a relatively small number of mental health service users are accessing direct payments and personal budgets, but the schemes are rapidly gaining in support and interest from mental health service users. They make it possible for service users to reassess their support needs in non-medicalised terms and secure the kind of assistance which they find helpful. This includes personal assistance; out of hours help; help with day-to-day tasks (like cooking, going out and shopping); counselling, advice and 'talking therapies'. Some service users are also putting parts of their budgets together to buy things together like training and recreational opportunities.

Self-run personal assistance schemes are not a panacea and they should be seen as an option, rather than the only approach available to service users. However, survivors receiving them report fewer inpatient hospital stays and the possibility of avoiding crises through having support in advance of their situation worsening.

If such schemes are to work for the wide range of mental health service users who are now entitled to them, then experience strongly indicates that local user-controlled organisations need to be established and properly funded and supported to offer the back-up, financial and technical support and advice to enable *every* service user (regardless of their experience and expertise) to run such a scheme without it being burdensome or difficult, even if they have a crisis or particularly bad time. The evidence from direct payments schemes for disabled people also highlights that the health of people receiving these schemes tends to improve and that they gain transferable skills which help them return to employment if they so wish. The transformative effects such schemes can have for people are summed up by Andy Smith, a mental health service user and strong advocate of them:

> In many respects people like me are the most persuasive argument in favour of self-directed support. Having used the funds to liberate myself and gain control and independence, the logical next step was to get myself educated to a level that would permit me to attempt to similarly improve the lives of other service users. Since my

involvement with SDS [self-directed support] both my
leisure and career options have multiplied. If it worked for
me, it might work for you.

Encouraging community development approaches

Mental health policy and provision have generally tended to
operate in relation to the individual. Initiatives which seek
to enable people to come together to achieve change and
support together, however, have a long and successful track
record in this field. These include, for example, the
pioneering work of truly democratic therapeutic
communities which offer therapeutic and group support; as
well as group work and group therapy. Community
development approaches, therefore, are likely to have a
particular contribution to offer in social approaches to
madness and distress. They make it possible to:

- reach out and involve a diverse range of service users
- challenge isolation by operating proactively rather than reactively
- engage with and understand service users in the context of their own communities (of locality, interest and identity)
- engage and reinforce the abilities and capacities of service users
- support collective working
- bring the strengths of mutual aid and support to bear in the context of collective action for change
- support self- and mutual empowerment

Community development approaches have frequently emphasised the importance of involvement and empowerment. They are especially helpful where service users and service user organisations employ them and have an effective say in how they are used.

The development of new roles and new approaches

Almost all the roles associated with mental health policy and practice have their origins in medicalised individual approaches to treatment and understanding. This is not a comment on their value or legitimacy. Mental health service users/survivors still most often comment on whether their psychiatrist, social worker or CPN (community psychiatric nurse) is a 'good' or a 'bad' one, according to the nature of the individual worker, rather than according to the inherent nature of the role. However, all the occupational and professional roles associated with the mental health system are more or less based on a model of 'mental illness'. This includes social work (despite its commitment to social approaches) and psychology – even if their analysis and interventions are different from those of mainstream psychiatry.

Now, with the advent of self-run services, complementary approaches, schemes for personal support and new approaches to self-management and self-support, it is particularly timely to explore new roles and new approaches to practice and occupational roles. This has already happened in the context of disability where new roles and services have been pioneered by the disabled people's movement. Here services not conceived in medicalised terms or in terms of rehabilitation or 'care' have developed over the last few years. This has resulted in new approaches to training as well as distinct new roles, usually based on the recruitment of people with direct experience of disability and impairment. This includes roles concerned with providing personal assistance, social and housing advice, peer advocacy and counselling and assessment. In some cases this has led to certificated training programmes as well as the emergence of recognised new roles.

This has also begun to happen in the field of mental health. However, it is a development which would now benefit from being taken forward in association with mental health service users and their organisations in a much more strategic and systematic way. There are already a number of emerging roles to build on and develop, for example:

- service user telephone helpline workers
- non-medicalised crisis and safe-house workers
- peer advocates
- advice workers
- employment and support workers
- non-medicalised support workers

Such roles need to be explored, training developed (and training materials produced) and schemes for accreditation established, to create a range of new roles alongside traditional mental health ones. There is also a place for developing new materials and input to support traditional roles (for example, in social work, occupational therapy and nursing) to address and include a social model of madness and distress and to explore its implications for the development of conventional practice.

Peter Campbell, founding member of the UK survivor movement, has summed up what a new approach to

support for mental health service users could look like and
how far it takes us from traditional models:

> What we need in future is support that is truly holistic.
> What we have now is a rhetorical commitment to holism
> but support remains restricted and dominated by a medical
> model approach. We need imaginative support which
> recognises the full humanity of people in mental distress.
> In particular, in future we should be seeing less
> compulsory care not more. It is that crisis will continue to
> be accompanied by unpleasant events like being picked up
> by the police and handcuffed into a police van, like
> restraint and solitary confinement. In these cases, what
> many people need is a chance to talk through the trauma
> not have it ignored. In general terms, whether there will be
> more therapy available or not, there definitely needs to be
> more human interaction going on, more talking and
> listening of a basic kind.
>
> It would be great to see the expertise of people with
> direct experience more available. This is partly to do with
> having more peer support workers but is also about
> ensuring that self-help groups are not squeezed out by
> professional-dominated support. Finally, the future will not
> look good for us unless we gain more choice and control
> over the support we want. These are key requirements.

In the present difficult economic times, Anne Beales, a
survivor who works for the mental health charity *Together*,
sums up the challenge we face:

> We need to face up to our fears about spending cuts in the
> mental health sector, supporting each other in resisting
> them, while putting into place alternative peer-led support

initiatives [services] which could radically change the landscape of mental health provision and even act as a lifeline to our very existence.

At its heart, peer support exists to benefit the individuals who engage with it, through building mutually beneficial relationships based on shared experience, trust and empathy. Evidence shows that these relationships provide people with self-help strategies that professionals may not be able to offer or even know about.

Peer support is by its very nature a community activity, and so it helps people break out of social exclusion. It also mirrors the language of the personalisation agenda, as self-directed and personal choice. Peer support also ticks the 'co-production' box as it cannot be done to or for us, and it begins to address our own agenda around what we (service users/survivors) mean by well-being.

Whilst we can't avoid the fact that any potential cuts will have a devastating impact on frontline services for people with mental health issues the service user movement should also recognise the opportunity to mobilise and promote the value of service user involvement as critical as well as cost-effective, because it *works*.

Chapter 10
Developing a new vision: Routes to achieving change

> Survivor research is developing a new foundation, just as
> users and survivors are in other areas, such as mental
> health policy, practice, education and anti-discrimination.
> This foundation is planting itself deep and cracking the
> bedrock of the most fundamental beliefs traditional mental
> health systems rest upon.[1]
>
> *Mary O'Hagan*

An alternative vision for mental health and a system of
support to go with it won't be achieved overnight. It won't
be achieved at all if is not supported and encouraged. It is
not enough to talk about encouraging managers or
'champions' to support change, as now tends to happen. If
that is all that happens, service users will be reliant on the
particular skills, quality and commitment of the leads in
their area, their mental health trust, their hospital and their
services. There will be the same concerns about the
patchiness of provision, with frequently expressed worries
about the 'postcode lottery' facing service users. They will
still be in essentially the same system. A radical survivor-led
strategy for an alternative mental health system is needed
that goes far beyond this.

At the heart of this must be 'an engine for change', with
a responsibility for advancing this aspiration. Central to this
is the contribution of the service user/survivor movement. If
we are to build on the commitment for change regularly

expressed by government, policymakers, progressive practitioners and service users, then the survivor movement will be the key starting point for it. It is difficult to see where else such a radical impulse will come from.

A number of key routes to change can be identified, if we are to advance the progressive principles and approaches to support set out in the last two chapters. These include:

- strengthening user-controlled organisations
- self-education and personal prevention
- societal education and prevention
- valuing user experience in the workforce
- continuity of support
- supporting user research and evaluation
- the improvement of quality based on developing user-defined standards
- ensuring a reliable and adequate income
- a transformed labour market – inclusive and less stressful

Strengthening user-controlled organisations

User-controlled organisations are the key active expression of the survivors and other service user movements. Independent, constituted user-controlled organisations have existed for nearly a generation. They have grown in numbers, effectiveness and influence in the last 10–15 years particularly. There are now local, regional, national and international organisations. They are greatly valued by many mental health service users. It has long been argued by disabled people and other service users that they provide the best route to developing personal empowerment and generating the impetus for progressive reform, both within and beyond the service system. Colin Barnes, Professor of Disability Studies and long-term disability activist, charts their origins in the disabled people's movement and the continuing uncertainties they face:

Since the 1970s, grass-roots user-controlled organisations, often referred to as Centres for Independent Living or CILs, have led the struggle for meaningful policies and services with which to eradicate the inequality and exclusion encountered by the overwhelming majority of disabled people, their families and service users generally. In 2000 there were over 80 user-controlled groups operating across the UK providing a range of independent living services with over half delivering direct payment-type support systems to disabled people, their families and other service users.

Yet despite recent government commitments to ensure that each local authority has a CIL-type organisation by the year 2010, local user-controlled service providers are closing at an alarming rate. Decades of under-funding and limited resources have meant that both local and national user-controlled agencies are severely disadvantaged in the increasingly competitive market for local and national contracts for independent living and direct payment-type services.

Hence access to meaningful local user-led support and direct payments/personal budgets-type schemes is a postcode lottery. All of which is directly at odds with recent government rhetoric espousing the need for independent living and the realisation of equal opportunities for disabled people and service users.

For mental health service users, user-controlled organisations have long provided a resource both for mutual aid and for positive social development. They play a crucial role in making possible what Judi Chamberlin called 'consciousness-raising', what the Latin American educator Paulo Friere called 'conscientization', what the US black civil rights movement called 'empowerment' and what some UK service user/survivor organisations now call 'capacity-building'. A crucial element of all these is the enhanced ability to see one's self in a new and positive light that makes the political connections with the world in which one lives. This is an ongoing process which makes it possible better to understand ourselves, the psychiatric system, how it sees and categorises us and how we can challenge this through recognising our potential for change.

Service users have repeatedly called for the adequate state funding of such independent organisations. We know that they can generate their own income through providing goods and services, but they need pump-priming with funding and other resources initially if they are to get off the ground and build their own and service users' capacity. Through outreach initiatives, they can provide one of the most effective routes to enabling broad and diverse involvement, as well as reaching out to include the views of service users who may not want to get actively involved. They play a central role in the thinking of service users, for example, providing the essential support and resources to enable the widest range of service users to access direct payments and personal budgets with confidence and without burden. Yet they are still both inadequately and insecurely funded. Frequently they rely on voluntary unpaid effort, without the essential infrastructure to maintain their effective operation, or are dependent on one service user worker, often working part-time. As a result, organisations frequently fold; in some areas there isn't such an organisation and service users involved are liable to burnout.

Bearing in mind the importance attached by government and services to user involvement, and the widespread view among service users that the existence of user-controlled organisations provides the crucial basis to enable it to happen and flourish, this is a fundamental problem. A strategic and systematic approach to the funding of user-controlled organisations is urgently required at national level. They are the bricks and mortar of the service user/survivor movement. Secure and adequate funding which enables organisations to plan and develop effectively is essential. Specific support for black and ethnic minority user-controlled organisations, as well as funding for outreach work with local black and minority ethnic communities are also essential.

As Colin Barnes makes clear, without such user-controlled organisations, the crucial user-led services and support which we discussed in the last chapter are likely to be marginalised:

> User-controlled services are quite different from traditional top-down provision run and controlled by professionals. Traditional top-down professionally led services are almost exclusively still organised around individualistic deficit/medical models of disability and disadvantage and delivered by a vast army of professional helpers. The end result is the gradual but inevitable disempowerment of the overwhelming majority of service users and their families.
>
> In contrast, user-controlled services were devised and developed by organisations controlled and run by service users. Today references to these services and the principles upon which they are based permeate almost all government and professionally led rhetoric on 'social care'.

Yet this has not been matched by meaningful policies and funding with which to develop further user-controlled service providers. Over the last decade there has been a significant decline in these organisations. Consequently control of the support systems for the growing numbers of service users remains, and is likely to remain so in the future, with professionally led agencies and large charities; the very opposite of what is needed.

Self-education and personal prevention

Most of us start by being personally ill-equipped to deal with madness and distress. Facing madness and distress for the first time is perhaps the worst time to try and equip yourself to deal with it. Crisis and vulnerability do not making learning easy. Frequently frightened, uncertain, confused and disorientated, people can find it very difficult to put into practice the usual skills and techniques that might help negotiate other major difficulties. We may not feel there is a problem, or we may be totally incapacitated by it because of all the terrifying folklore we have unconsciously learned about 'going mad' and being 'mentally ill'. The people around us are likely to be just as frightened and in just as vulnerable a position. It is difficult to overstate the power of the fear of going mad in societies like ours – however rarely such matters may be discussed.

This is why it is important that madness and distress are subjects which we can learn (and talk) about (with reliable, independent information) from our earliest days. There is an important role here for schools and education services, from primary and pre-school onwards. Children are expected to learn how to look after themselves physically. Little of the same attention is paid to equipping them to maintain their mental well-being, although childhood and adolescence can be times of particular difficulty. There is not just the task of supporting people with helpful learning. Children are bombarded with 'mentalist' imagery. It is important to challenge conventional negative stereotypes of 'mad people' that are as commonplace on children's TV and in comic and kids' magazines as in adult media (sometimes though, coexisting with really helpful first-hand accounts by children and young people who have experienced distress).

Education about mental health issues should be a central component in the national curriculum and specifically in citizenship education, from primary school onwards. It should address the whole range of issues, from rights and stigma to support and self-management. This is a process that needs to permeate all aspects of society, opposing the mentalist imagery and assumptions that still predominate. Some television soaps have begun to address issues of disability in an anti-discriminatory and inclusive way. The same has yet to happen effectively for mental health issues. There is also an important role here for employers, supporting people with experience as mental health service users to join the workforce and spreading the word that they have a contribution to make in it.

There is now a vast amount of clear, helpful information available about mental health matters. But madness and distress are still so much taboo subjects and the dominant (popular as well as professional) discussion about them is so bound up in fear and internalised oppression, that it is still hard for many people routinely to turn to these. We all need to be equipped to recognise the early warning signs, to have a better understanding of what might be happening. But this is not a task that should be left to the individual. Just as we are finding out more about diet and alcohol use, sports injuries and preparation for retirement, so more needs to be done at an infrastructural level to equip individuals to be able to recognise, acknowledge and respond to madness, distress and using mental health services as potential aspects of all our lives.

Societal education and prevention

Health promotion and education have so far mainly been framed in individualist terms, aiming to get the individual to adapt to more healthy ways of living. Clearly this can be helpful in the context of mental health too, but it is not enough on its own. A broader social approach is also needed, which takes account not only of individual experience, but also the effects of social oppressions and barriers on people's mental (as well as physical) well-being. We know that disempowerment, discrimination, oppression and inequality all play their part in engendering distress. As a result there are particular problems for people at undue risk of facing such oppression, like women and black and minority ethnic communities.

We also know that pressures from poor working conditions, poverty, and social and family breakdown can all contribute to personal distress and breakdown. To provide the basis for prevention and education at societal levels, it would be helpful to identify the elements that are likely to have damaging effects on people's psychological well-being in a more coherent and systematic way; to monitor and audit them and to explore ways of minimising damaging effects. This should be a routine task of social policy, undertaking cost/benefit analyses of existing policies and arrangements, as well as new developments in public policy, in order to evaluate their implications and likely impact on madness and distress.

In this way, it would be possible to develop indices which can help to avoid and reduce the incidence of distress. The financial costs of madness and distress are massive. Mental health policy and provision are costly, even though for many service users they are experienced as negative and of very limited help. Public policy needs to be subjected to broader, more rigorous evaluation that takes account of the human and financial costs generated by the creation and perpetuation of distress. The indices emerging from such an exercise are likely to provide a more helpful basis for informing and interpreting the economics of policy, which takes account of the frequently neglected psychological costs of market and state policies.

There is also one specific area for priority attention: the important negative role which parts of the media play in the construction of madness and distress. Mental health service users identify stigma as one of the fundamental problems they face. Stigma perpetuates hostility, misunderstanding and exclusion. It is time that enforceable codes of conduct were developed in association with service users and introduced to regulate the media's presentation of 'mental health' issues and mental health service users. Mentalist language like 'loony', 'nutter', 'schizo' and the rest need to be challenged, as should the tendency of the tabloid press to 'racialise' issues of violence in relation to mental health service users. This is one specific area for regulation and change which could have a rapid impact on public understanding.

In recent years growing attention has been paid to the negative stereotyping and stigma associated with mental health issues. There have been costly, large scale anti-stigma campaigns, which have tended to focus on 'public education'. It is debatable how much good they can do, as long as politicians, policymakers and the media themselves continue to stereotype and scapegoat mental health service users/survivors as 'benefits scroungers' and malingerers, as we have increasingly seen happen in recent years. Such powerful opinion-formers, individuals and institutions need to be prioritised as candidates for re-education if madness and distress are truly to come out of the closet and no longer feel like taboo subjects.

Valuing user experience in the workforce

There is still a strongly ambivalent attitude to the experience of using mental health services in health and social care services. Some workers report that while these are policy areas where greater understanding of such issues might be expected, often their experience has been the opposite and conventional commercial organisations have shown better understanding, more supportive attitudes and responses. People who have experienced distress while working in the health and social care sectors frequently report negative responses; being sidelined and seen as no longer suitable for promotion and being encouraged to leave. Some people are reluctant to be open about their experience of distress for fear of discrimination and negative repercussions.

At the same time, as a result of pioneering initiatives and growing recognition of the importance of paid employment for the self-esteem and well-being of mental health service users, increasing efforts are now being made to support the involvement of people with experience as mental health service users in the health care workforce. These have demonstrated the capacity of a wide range of people with such experience to make an effective contribution which also has major personal benefits.

If such developments are to expand and service workers' experiences of distress are to be more positively addressed, health and social care policy and services must be encouraged to develop a more positive approach to direct experience of mental distress in their workforce. This will not only make it more possible that the most appropriate and supportive response can be made to such experience. It will also make it possible for people with direct experience of distress to make an even greater contribution as service providers – something which service users value. It is important that this development is systematically developed and carefully monitored and evaluated to ensure that people with experience as service users have the same opportunities as other workers, are not ghettoised in lower status (or 'user involvement') work, have positive career opportunities and that employment opportunities are primarily developed to meet the needs of service user workers rather than the organisational interests of the service system. As in other areas of employment, it will mean re-examining employment practices to ensure they are flexible and supportive, minimising rather than exacerbating emotional distress and occupational stress. While anti-discrimination legislation is not strong in the UK, it does offer some basis for challenging discrimination and improving survivors' experience in employment, for example, through negotiating and agreeing 'reasonable adjustments' under the Disability Discrimination Act to enable them to work on more equal terms.

Continuity of support

The large-scale adoption of a 'mental illness'-based approach to distress has meant that responses have tended to be framed in terms of 'treatment'. Some diagnostic categories have tended to be seen as long lasting or even permanent and 'incurable'. Generally though, as with physical illness, the assumption is that the purpose of mental health provision is to provide 'treatment' in order that people can 'get better'. This has tended to mean that where people's situations are seen to improve; where they feel they are more able to do things, they have got over a crisis or 'bad time', then support is reduced or removed.

This is the routine experience of many mental health service users and it is one which they frequently find very unhelpful and destabilising. While getting back into the routine of life, getting a job and having more control over their lives are taken to mean that 'treatment' is no longer needed, many service users feel that they need support at that point just as much as before (sometimes more). This model of providing support when things are bad and removing it when service users are seen to be 'better' is likely to gain even greater force now with the widespread adoption of a 'recovery' model in Britain, as we discussed in the last chapter. This model is firmly based on a 'mental illness' approach to distress and reflects its shortcomings.

As has been said, it is likely to be much more helpful to think of support for mental health service users in similar terms to the way it is understood for other people identified as disabled. Here there is an understanding that what people need is support, and that while the nature of that support may change, the need for it may be long lasting or indeed constant, if they are to function fully and live 'independently'. Mental health service users may still need support when they are back in employment and have their own informal support arrangements in place. This should not be seen as a reason for removing or reducing such support. This is the equivalent of taking away a disabled person's wheelchair and other mobility aids because they are achieving their potential. Service users' definitions of their support needs should be central to policy and practice and simplistic assumptions based on 'getting well' need to be subjected to fundamental review.

Supporting user research and evaluation

In just the last few years, a radical new idea has entered research and evaluation. It now has the support of government, many statutory and non-statutory funders, progressive researchers, research organisations – and service users and their organisations. Key new organisations, like Involve (formerly Consumers in NHS Research) and the Joseph Rowntree Foundation, a major independent funder of social policy research, are seeking to take the idea forward in health and social care research. It is meant to underpin the work of the government's Mental Health Research Network and its National Institute for Health Research. This is the idea and practice of service user involvement in research. The aim is to ensure that the viewpoint of service users is included in the production and development of research. The goal is to take account of service users' perspectives and understandings, as well as those of other stakeholders. Service users may be involved in all aspects of research projects, from identifying the research focus and question(s), to undertaking research, data collection, collation, analysis and writing up, as well as dissemination and follow-up action. They are also encouraged to contribute to all aspects of research more generally, from commissioning and peer review, to setting priorities and developing methods and methodologies.[2]

Service users and their organisations have not only got involved in mainstream health and social care research. They have also developed their own 'user-controlled' and 'emancipatory' research approaches. Such research emphasises a new, more equal process of undertaking research, with more equal relationships between service users and researchers; an emphasis on supporting the empowerment of service users and research not only to extend knowledge, but to lead to broader social change. A wide range of projects, big and small, are now being carried out in this way, exploring issues, creating new knowledge and making possible broader change in line with service users'/survivors' priorities, rights and needs.[3]

A growing number of 'user researchers' are now undertaking research, including both quantitative and qualitative research, and small scale and increasingly larger projects. As yet only a tiny proportion of commissioned health and social care research comes from service users, but this is beginning to have an impact on knowledge production, policy and practice. The development of user involvement in research and service user research are helping to provide more relevant and inclusive research and evaluation, which can provide a better knowledge base for mental health policy and practice. Both have a key role to play in monitoring, evaluating and developing more social approaches to distress. They make it possible for knowledge production to be a truly collaborative process. More work needs to be done on supporting and evaluating such research approaches if they are to fulfil this potential.

Developing quality, embracing user-defined standards

There is now a growing policy emphasis on and political interest in improving quality in public services. This has extended to health and welfare, including mental health services. It is reflected in the creation of national service frameworks, including that for mental health, which lay down standards and goals for policy and provision, as well as a more general preoccupation with standards, 'targets' and 'regulation'. The emphasis on standards in recent years has been reflected in the development of a wide range of measures, including performance indicators (for agencies and staff) and quality and outcome measures. This has been linked with an increasing concern with audit, review and measurement.

Critics have argued that a preoccupation with measurement does not necessarily lead to an improvement in quality and indeed may have the opposite effect, leading to increasing bureaucratisation. But there is another issue, which has less often been raised. Such standards and criteria for quality and quality improvement have generally been based on managerial and professional criteria. However there is evidence to show that what service users want and prioritise does not always reflect the concerns and priorities of service providers and policymakers.

Service user-controlled organisations, like Shaping Our Lives, have sought to explore and develop related ideas of user-defined measures and standards. Here service users identify what they mean by improved quality, priorities and measures of good services. If the aim is to develop support and services which match the preferences (of the diverse range) of service users, then it is essential that standards and measures also draw upon the views of service users and that service users are effectively included in the process of establishing such measures and making use of them. If the aim is to change the value base of mental health services and move to a (social) model of policy and provision that represents a departure from traditional approaches, then it is especially important for service users and their organisations to be centrally involved in the conceptualisation and development of quality strategy.

Ensuring a reliable and adequate income

As I write this, government has embarked upon another major campaign of 'welfare reform'. This has been a feature of modern UK social policy. It has hit mental health service users/survivors particularly hard. This time it has mainly been framed in terms of 'waging war on benefit cheats'. Spearheaded by the media, it has generated a strong populist response, strengthening hostility against people on benefits. Even before this campaign, politicians were talking of getting 'a million people off incapacity benefits' in the UK. This has especially targeted mental health service users, whose general lack of wheelchairs, hearing and other aids, visible impairments and physical health conditions has long meant that their difficulties have not been well understood. They have faced particular difficulties in securing disability benefits and have tended to be the first to have them withdrawn. Medical testing has also become increasingly harsh, subjecting mental health service users/survivors to more frequent and more intimidating checks and reviews. Levels of fear and anxiety have been raised and survivors' worries that some people will be driven to commit suicide as a result have been raised and already in some publicly reported cases, seem to have been justified.

What is needed is a reliable and flexible system to ensure mental health service users a secure and adequate income. Arrangements must take account of fluctuations in people's situation and enable them to move in and out of employment without disadvantage, if that is an option for them. There has long been discussion of the 'benefit' or 'poverty trap', which means that many people are fearful of coming off benefits because they cannot earn as much in employment. This problem needs to be recognised as related not to the low motivation of service users, but to the high cost of housing and the generally low wages that mental health service users are able to earn because of the discrimination they face as well as the difficulties created by their mental health problems. These larger social problems will need to be resolved to overcome these difficulties and in the long term this will require major changes in housing and a more flexible, inclusive and socially responsible employment market.

A transformed labour market – inclusive and less stressful

Work is important in all our lives. Paid work is how many people have a sense of contribution and purpose, where they meet people, make friends and form relationships and how they constructively occupy much of their time.

The statistics show that people who are long-term users of mental health services are much less likely to be in employment than other people and that they are likely to be concentrated in lower paid, less desirable, poorer quality jobs. They are not valued as members of the labour market and can expect to be seen as having less to offer it. This adds to problems of poverty and social isolation. Getting a job is frequently seen as the solution to the problem, particularly by powerful people and policymakers, who express concern about a 'dependency culture' and want to cut public spending on health and welfare benefits. But while employment is presented as a panacea for all, including mental health service users/survivors, it actually raises a whole set of its own problems, particularly given the direction that it has taken in recent years, with increasing economic globalisation and insecurity.

Old arrangements of 'jobs for life', secure pensions and improved working conditions resulting from many years of collective struggle have been replaced for most by insecure employment, deferred retirement, uncertainty about the future and poorer 'terms and conditions' of work. The evidence shows that economic inequality has greatly increased in the UK and social mobility has been significantly reduced. People generally are working longer hours; some have to have more than one job to make ends meet. There have been growing concerns about the 'work/ life balance', people having to spend more time commuting to work and having less time for their family, friends and children. Despite the introduction of the 'minimum wage', wages have been driven down and more and more people have had to be subsidised by state benefits and tax rebates and credits when in work.

Thus while mental health service users/survivors can expect to be under increasing pressure to get a job, the kind of work and wages available to them are as likely to add to their mental health problems and insecurity as offer any solutions. The instrumental nature of employment and the labour market means that both are increasingly being seen as major sources of mental health problems in our society. They play an ambiguous role, as much generating psychological problems of distress as countering them.

If employment is truly to serve a positive purpose for mental health service users/survivors then its antisocial elements must be challenged; it will need to become less discriminatory and more flexible to accommodate them, their needs and their potential contribution. Service users will need greater support to access meaningful training and education that is geared to qualification and improving their employment skills and prospects. At the same time, worthwhile alternatives need to be available for service users for whom even more flexible formal employment continues to be too difficult.

Postscript
A broader view and next steps

> We must not let ourselves be reduced to arbitrary
> constructions ... we must not let someone else tell our
> stories and have control over who we become.[1]
> *US survivor and activist Sherry Mead*

At the beginning of this book, I said that fear was a key
word for me in my experience of madness, distress and the
service systems I came to encounter. But there's also one
other word that keeps recurring for me. That word is
'isolation'. It takes many expressions. People experiencing
mental health problems frequently become isolated. There is
talk of 'social isolation', 'social exclusion', loneliness and
'loners'. Psychiatric services have their own significant
isolating effects, because of the stigma and stereotyping that
go with them and their own segregating nature. But there is
another key sense in which this word isolation is important.
There is a strong tendency for madness and distress and
mental health service users/survivors to be considered and
talked about in isolation. This is as if they were a separate
problem and a separate group of people. 'Experts' often put
narrow boundaries around this field of discussion, treating it
as a specialist focus of professional or research concern. Yet
while we know that different things affect people in
different ways and that not everyone seems to run the same
risk of entering the psychiatric system, there is no doubt
that there are real links between what happens to people in

their wider world and madness and distress. The latter can only truly be understood in terms of us and our relation with our worlds.

Challenging a maddening world

As sociologists have long told us (but many psychiatrists still find difficult to understand) life is largely about the interactions between individuals and the wider world they inhabit. We may not know what the balance is between 'nature' and 'nurture' – between our individual make-up and what happens to us – in shaping the person we become – but as John Donne said centuries ago 'no man is an island'. We are all affected by society. What each of us does may have a bearing on it. And society has a bearing – generally much greater – on each of us. Our stories are essentially about the intersection of our individual biography with history – what happens more widely.

But I want to highlight something else here that is crucially important for all – our mental well-being. This is the degree to which we live in a 'maddening' world. By this I mean the extent to which societies and the wider world are supportive of our mental and physical well-being – it is difficult truly to separate the two – or create obstacles in the way of them. In my view our world is one that is very maddening, although of course this is not true equally for everyone. Some people, in some situations, some communities, some countries and some parts of the world, are particularly exposed. Let me say a bit more about what I mean when I talk of a 'maddening world'. While we can expect as mental health service users/survivors to be told off for being 'different', we also often have a sense that we live in a world that is itself inherently irrational and a world which frequently drives people to madness and distress.

While people always say that what they want most in the world is peace, what characterises it constantly are war and conflict. While in recent years mental health service users/ survivors have come under growing attack for being threatening and dangerous – for their association with homicides – ours is a world that in other contexts celebrates the military, has exhibitions of its killing machines and at particular times expects men to carry out orders to kill in war, unless they can offer convincing 'conscientious objections' to doing so.

Such wars are constant and truly on a global scale, between nationals, ethnic groups, tribes, ideologies, religions and world powers. War is an extreme example of the maddening nature of society. While we are generally taught from childhood that to kill is murder, killing for our country has long been made a large-scale exception. More money is spent on war and weapons globally than anything else. There has only been one year since the end of the last world war in 1945 when a British soldier has not been killed in fighting. The UK's most successful industry is the arms trade. The manufacture of weapons and their use is one of the greatest, if not the greatest polluters of the environment, yet we focus instead for a greener future on campaigns against the use of plastic shopping bags.

Modern war creates many more civilian than military casualties and high among these are psychiatric casualties. War literally drives many people mad. It is also no respecter of age. Children, older people and other adults are all exposed to its destructive effects. One feature of recent conflicts has been the use of 'child soldiers' as well as conscripted adults. War is strongly associated with madness and distress. This is most often discussed in psychiatrised terms of 'post traumatic stress disorder' (PTSD). It is difficult to see, however, how a 'normal' human reaction to danger, terror and the prospect of injury and death can be constructed as a 'disorder'. It is interesting to note that the number of UK combatants who committed suicide following the Falklands war of the 1980s is now greater than the number who were actually killed in action. Grim statistics about the scale of long-term mental health problems following involvement in conflicts are increasingly emerging and these take no account of the additional mental suffering endured by others as a result of people's personalities being changed through war and through the effects of large-scale impairment, loss and bereavement.

War is just an extreme example of the topsy-turvy nature of our world and its maddening effects. It is also a world where globalisation and the inadequately regulated activities of multinational companies and massive corporations are praised and valued, yet these are closely associated with the most terrible damage to the environment, animal and plant life and the sustainability of the planet. Ours is a society where people can be and are fined for dropping litter and sent to prison for not sending their children to school. Yet only a tiny proportion of women who are raped ever see their rapist convicted and sentences against rapists and child sexual offenders can be minimal, for example, compared with those handed out for robbery, drug offences and even non-violent animal rights protest. Yet we know that sex offences against women and children, for example, can have a devastating and enduring effect on the mental health of those who are victimised and can be the reason why they end up as mental health service users and are at greater than usual risk of committing suicide.

We know that all the following are closely associated with madness and distress:

- insecurity
- powerlessness
- oppression and abuse
- discrimination
- exclusion
- material want

We also know that they continue to be commonplace consequences of the unequal distribution of power, status, value and resources in our world and our society.

Further insights into the relationship between the wider world and the individual are offered by people's widespread reliance on mind-altering drugs. The scale of people's reliance and dependence on both prescription and illegal drugs does raise the question of what is it about the world we live in that leads so many people to do this. Carolyn Anderson, commenting particularly on what she sees as the relation between abuse and 'schizophrenia', also highlights a negative relation she sees between one drug and people's madness and distress. At the heart of her comments is the relation between people's distress and their wider experience in society.

> I believe there are two main factors that account for the onset of schizophrenia. One is the long-term use of drugs such as cannabis and the other is long-term abuse in both early childhood and in later years. The abuse can take many forms such as sexual abuse, physical abuse, verbal abuse from a sibling, friend or family member or bullying. All children need to be loved and nurtured and if they are deprived of this basic need, the effects can be quite traumatic.

The trauma of long-term abuse seems to stay in the subconscious and it may not surface until years later in the form of mental illness. It may be that stress plays a major part in all of this and that the early trauma, because it has not been dealt with and discussed fully through talking therapy, may affect how a person reacts to stress which then builds up until their brain can no longer cope with it and a person is then pushed into psychosis and then into full-blown schizophrenia.

My belief is based on the many friends and service users I know who suffer from schizophrenia and whose lives have been shattered by its devastating effects. Many of them have become fairly stable and are able to cope with their illness, but for others the nightmare goes on.

It would of course be wrong to assume that if the world became a less cruel, abusive and oppressive, more equal and accepting place, that we would put an end to madness and distress. There will always be bereavements, failures in love and relationships, disappointments, tragedies and other difficulties overshadowing people's lives and mental states. But it is difficult not to think that, if we lived in a world more guided by concern for people's well-being, then the scale of problems they faced would be reduced.

There have been some recent shifts in government thinking and policies which reflect some recognition of these issues. For example, there has been more official talk about people's 'happiness' and suggestions that more than material well-being is needed to make such happiness possible. But such discussions always come unstuck because of the lack of agreement there tends to be about what 'happiness' is and whether it can or should be legislated for. Another political approach has been to talk of 'total place', where the aim is for all policies to be linked and directed at maximising local communities' and citizens' well-being and cohesion. But while the rhetoric has become more commonplace, the thrust of policy continues to be to cut local amenities, support services and public transport and to give an increasing role to centralising policies and large commercial organisations preoccupied with profit and competition. A third example has been government's 'New Horizons: Better mental well-being programme'. This has had the aim of improving the 'mental well-being of all'. However, mental health service users/survivors have expressed concern both that it has not been linked with any necessary wider changes in public policy and that it may divert resources from the inadequate mental health services available for current service users.

We should not lose sight of the connections that there may be between people's madness and distress and the nature of the world and society they live in. We must always include the latter in the equation and work for big change as well as for change within ourselves. We must challenge the maddening nature of society and seek to lessen it. This is what Peter Campbell, one of the founders of the UK survivors' movement, has to say about a 'maddening world':

> A less maddening world would have got rid of all the negative preconceptions about madness. This would be connected to a much wider and more open debate about the true nature of madness in which all sections of society took part on a level playing field. Misconceptions about the violence and threat posed by 'the mad' would go out the window as would the critically disempowering assumption that the mad have no insight and cannot be trusted to know what their best interests are.
>
> Of course, it would be great to live in a world that was less stressful, where people were less isolated, where we

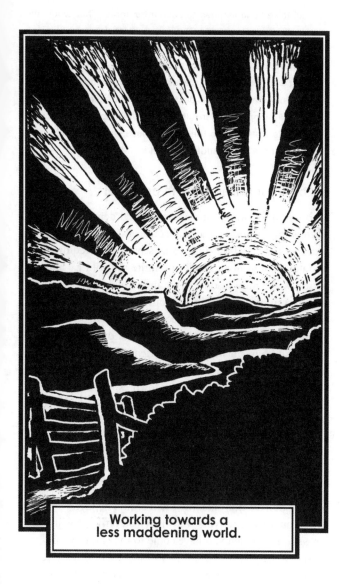

Working towards a
less maddening world.

all talked and listened to each other more. That would be a less maddening world. But equally important would be a transformed attitude to difference. Not a denial of difference, for in certain respects the mad are different, but a tolerance of difference and a revaluing that says, 'Yes, we are different but different and equal not different and inferior. Not alien.' If we could reshape madness and people's attitude to the mad in these ways, that might make for a less maddening world.

Both the political and the personal

Madness and distress truly are issues that demand we address the broadest structural concerns and the most intimate aspects of our individual selves. They require that we take account of and seek to reunite the political and the personal. We must also keep the individual and the person in the front of our thinking. In our efforts to bring about positive change in line with people's rights and self-defined needs, we should always be reflecting our own understandings, on what our experience has been, what we have found helpful and what we have valued from others.

What have I learned from my own experience of madness and distress? It is a question I ask myself as many others may ask the same of themselves. I have learned that to some extent at least I can cope. There is much to cope with in this life and world. I rely on the support of others. I have been fortunate to have it. I have good and bad times. Sometimes I feel I have achieved something in my life. At others I don't. I don't assume I will always be OK. Many of us call ourselves survivors. But truly you only know if you have survived when you have come to the end of your journey. I have known a number of mental health service users/survivors who have felt that they had to end their lives. But I feel all of them achieved a lot and that their struggles were worthwhile.

I have learned some basic lessons which I have found helpful. Others may have their own pet lists. This is mine:

- one thing at a time
- try and live day by day, one step at a time
- don't anticipate troubles and problems
- try not to take things too personally
- give yourself the same advice you'd give others
- try not to judge others – this is the basis for all kindness and wisdom
- look for the good in others
- all things pass – including the bad things
- you can do it, just as others have done it before you
- don't feel ground down by your failures. Everyone has them. Don't beat yourself up. Try and learn from them
- doing things with others is the best way
- together, even if on a modest scale, we can make a difference, we can make things better
- by understanding ourselves better, we can better understand the world
- by understanding ourselves better, we are better placed to change the world

I've also learned some lessons from my experience in the psychiatric and benefits system:

- we are all different
- our experience of madness and distress can be very

different. Things I have dreaded, for example, others seem to have no problem with and vice versa. But we all face similar barriers and difficulties

• no one is less than me. I am not less than them

• whatever anybody else thinks of me, I have a right to hold to who and what I think I am

• madness and distress take many forms. Experiencing any of them makes it more possible to understand that of someone else

• we can get real help and support from others. But the people we can feel closest too and who offer the most natural understanding and mutual aid are people who have 'been there' like us

To make progress we will need to understand ourselves. We will be helped to do that through working with others and in turn that greater self-understanding will strengthen what we can do together. We will need to form alliances, particularly with other people and groups who face discrimination and oppression. This is where our strength and potential will lie. We will need to develop ways of working that include people facing some of the biggest personal and social barriers, people who find it difficult to leave their homes, difficult to communicate and to be with others. Since our way of making change is from the bottom up and begins with working for change within ourselves, we will always be able to make progress. There is no limit to where that may take us. Wherever we get, we can have real confidence that we will know ourselves and others and feel better about both than we would ever otherwise have done. There is a better place and we have a key part to play in achieving it.

Endnotes

Foreword

1. See this volume, Postscript p. 123.

Introduction

1. Sweeney, A (2009) Mickey Mouse scans? In A Sweeney, P Beresford, A Faulkner, M Nettle & D Rose (Eds) (2009) *This Is Survivor Research* (pp 165–6). Ross-on-Wye: PCCS Books.

Chapter 2

1. Page xiv in Chamberlin, J (1988) *On Our Own: Patient-controlled alternatives to the mental health system*. London: MIND.

2. Page 272 in Heller, T & Walsh, M (2009) Challenges for practice. Introduction. In J Reynolds, R Muston, T Heller, J Leach, M McCormick, J Wallcraft & M Walsh (Eds) *Mental Health Still Matters* (pp 271–6). Basingstoke: Palgrave/Macmillan.

3. DRC (2006) *Equal Treatment: Closing the gap* (Report of formal investigation). London: Disability Rights Commission.

4. American Psychiatric Association (2000) *Diagnostic and Statistical Manual of Mental Disorders* (4th ed, text revision) (DSM-IV-TR). Washington, DC: American Psychiatric Association.

Chapter 3

1. Pages 3 and 7 in Wallcraft, J & Nettle, M (2009) History, context and language. In J Wallcraft, B Schrank & M Amering (Eds) *Handbook of Service User Involvement in Mental Health Research* (pp 1–11). World Psychiatric Association, Chichester: Wiley-Blackwell.

Chapter 4

1. Page 166 in Donskoy, A-L (2009) Benefit of the doubt. In A Sweeney, P Beresford, A Faulkner, M Nettle & D Rose (Eds) *This Is Survivor Research* (pp 166–7). Ross-on-Wye: PCCS Books.

2. Page 218 in Campbell, P (1996) The history of the user movement in the United Kingdom. In T Heller, J Reynolds, R Gomm, R Muston & S Pattison (Eds) *Mental Health Matters* (pp 218–25). Basingstoke: Macmillan, in association with the Open University.

3. Campbell, P (2009) The service user/survivor movement. In J Reynolds, R Muston, T Heller, J Leach, M McCormick, J Wallcraft & M Walsh (Eds) *Mental Health Still Matters* (pp 46–52). Basingstoke: Palgrave/Macmillan.

4. See page 49 in Campbell, P (2009) See note 3.

5. Page 48 in Campbell, P (2009) See note 3.

6. Jordan, T & Lent, A (Eds) (1999) *Storming the Millennium: The new politics of change.* London: Lawrence and Wishart.

7. Lent, A (2002) *British Social Movements since 1945: Sex, colour, peace and power.* Basingstoke: Palgrave/Macmillan.

8. Oliver, M (1996) *Understanding Disability: From theory to practice.* Basingstoke: Macmillan.

9. Shera, W & Wells, LM (Eds) (1999) *Empowerment Practice in Social Work: Developing richer conceptual foundations.* Toronto: Canadian Scholars' Press.

10. Page 48 in Campbell, P (2009). See note 3.

Chapter 5

1. Page 39 in Wallcraft, J, Read, J & Sweeney, A (2003) *On Our Own Terms: Users and survivors of mental health services working together for support and change.* London: Sainsbury Centre for Mental Health.

2. Howley, D (2009) Result of a bipolar endgame should not be a lottery. *Society Guardian,* 26 August, p 2.

3. Gomm, R (2009) Mental health and inequality. In J Reynolds, R Muston, T Heller, J Leach, M McCormick, J Wallcraft, & M Walsh (Eds) *Mental Health Still Matters* (pp 96–109). Basingstoke: Palgrave/Macmillan.

4. Sayce, L (2000) *From Psychiatric Patient to Citizen: Overcoming discrimination and social exclusion.* Basingstoke: Macmillan.

5. Gomm, 2009. See note 3.

6. McFarlane, L (1998) *Diagnosis: Homophobic – The experiences of lesbians, gay men and bisexuals in mental health services.* London: PACE (Promoting Lesbian and Gay Health and Wellbeing).

7. Busfield, J (2006) Mental disorder and human rights. In L Morris (Ed) *Human Rights: Sociological perspectives.* London and New York: Routledge.

8. King, M & McKeown, E (2003) Mental health and social well-being of gay men, lesbians and bisexuals in England and Wales. *The British Journal of Psychiatry, 183,* 552–8.

9. Bent, KN & McGilvy, J (2006) When a partner dies: Lesbian widows. *Issues in Mental Health Nursing, 27*(5), 447–59.

10. Rivers, I & Carragher, DJ (2003) Social-developmental factors affecting lesbian and gay youth: A review of cross-national research findings. *Children and Society, 17*(5), 374–85.

11. Pages 72–3 in Staddon, P (2005) Labelling out: The personal account of an ex-alcoholic lesbian feminist. In E Ettorre (Ed), *Making Lesbians Visible in the Substance Use Field.* New York: Haworth Press.

12. Beresford, P (2000) *Our Voice in Our Future: Mental health issues.* London: Shaping Our Lives/National Institute for Social Work.

13. Browne, D (2009) Black communities, mental health and the criminal justice system. In J Reynolds, R Muston, T Heller, J Leach, M McCormick, J Wallcraft & M Walsh (Eds), *Mental Health Still Matters* (pp 167–73). Basingstoke: Palgrave/Macmillan.

14. Page 3 in Morris, J (Ed) (1996) *Encounters with Strangers: Feminism and disability.* London: The Women's Press.

Chapter 6
1. Page 170 in Webb, D (2009) Being a survivor researcher helps me survive. In A Sweeney, P Beresford, A Faulkner, M Nettle & D Rose (Eds) (2009) *This Is Survivor Research* (pp 170–1). Ross-on-Wye: PCCS Books.

Chapter 7
1. Page 45 in Oliver, M (1996) *Understanding Disability: From theory to practice.* Basingstoke: Macmillan.

2. Beresford, P, Nettle, M & Perring, R (2010) *Towards a Social Model of Madness and Distress.* York: Joseph Rowntree Foundation.

3. Oliver, M (1996) *Understanding Disability: From theory to practice.* Basingstoke: Macmillan.

4. Oliver, M & Barnes, C (1998) *Disabled People and Social Policy: From exclusion to inclusion.* Harlow: Longman.

5. Thomas, C (2007) *Sociologies of Disability and Illness: Contested ideas in disability studies and medical sociology.* Basingstoke: Palgrave Macmillan.

6. Thomas, 2007. See n. 5.

7. Beresford, P, Nettle, M & Perring, R (2010) See n. 2.

8. Ramon, S & Williams, JE (Eds) (2005) *Mental Health at the Crossroads: The promise of the psychosocial approach.* Guildford: Ashgate.

9. Tew, J (Ed) (2005) *Social Perspectives in Mental Health: Developing social models to understand and work with mental distress.* London: Jessica Kingsley.

10. Beresford et al., 2010. See n. 2.

Chapter 8
1. Page 81 in Wallcraft, J, Read, J & Sweeney, A (2003) *On Our Own Terms: Users and survivors of mental health services working together for support and change.* London: Sainsbury Centre for Mental Health.

2. Morris, J (1993) *Independent lives? Community care and disabled people.* Basingstoke: Macmillan.

3. Campbell, J & Oliver, M (1996) *Disability Politics: Understanding our past, changing our future.* London: Routledge.

4. Morris, J (2004) Community care: A disempowering framework. *Disability & Society, 19*(5), 427–42.

5. ODI (2008) *The Independent Living Strategy: A cross-government strategy about independent living for disabled people.* London: Office for Disability Issues.

6. Pilgrim, D (2008) 'Recovery' and current mental health policy. *Chronic Illness, 4,* 295–304.

7. Turner-Crowson, J & Wallcraft, J (2002) The recovery vision for mental health services and research: A British perspective. *Psychiatric Rehabilitation Journal, 25*(3), 245–54.

8. Wilson, A & Beresford, P (2000) 'Anti-oppressive practice': Emancipation or appropriation? *British Journal of Social Work, 30,* 553–73.

9. Pages 31–42 in Wallcraft, J, Read, J & Sweeney, A (2003). See n.1.

Chapter 9

1. Front cover of Chamberlin, J (1988) *On Our Own: Patient-controlled alternatives to the mental health system.* London: MIND.

2. Page xiii in Chamberlin, 1988. See n. 1.

3. Page 18 in Chamberlin, 1988. See n. 1.

4. Chamberlin, 1988. See n. 1.

5. Page 18 in Chamberlin, 1988. See n. 1.

6. Barnes, C & Mercer, G (2006) *Independent Futures: Creating user-led disability services in a disabling society.* Bristol: Policy Press in association with the British Association of Social Workers.

7. Page 6 in Chamberlin, 1988. See n. 1.

8. Page 68 in Chamberlin, 1988. See n. 1.

9. Page 94 in Chamberlin, 1988. See n. 1.

10. Page 106 in Chamberlin, 1988. See n. 1.

Chapter 10

1. Page i, Foreword, in Sweeney, A, Beresford, P, Faulkner, A, Nettle, M & Rose, D (Eds) (2009) *This Is Survivor Research*. Ross-on-Wye: PCCS Books.

2. Wallcraft, J, Schrank, B & Amering, M (Eds) (2009) *Handbook of Service User Involvement in Mental Health Research.* World Psychiatric Association, Chichester: Wiley-Blackwell.

3. Sweeney, A, Beresford, P, Faulkner, A, Nettle, M & Rose, D, 2009. See n. 1.

Postscript

1. US survivor and activist Sherry Mead, cited in *Advocacy Update, European Network of (ex) Users and Survivors of Psychiatry, 2010, 1*(1), 3.

Contacts and resources

This is not a complete list. We have included telephone numbers or postal addresses where available for readers without internet access. Most of these groups do not have the resources to respond to individual requests for advice and support regarding treatment.

European Network of (ex)Users and Survivors of Psychiatry
http://www.enusp.org/

Hearing Voices Network
http://www.hearing-voices.org/
0144 271 8210

Intervoice: An international group for voice hearers
http://www.intervoiceonline.org/

Mad Pride   http://madpride.org.uk/

Mind
http://www.mind.org.uk/   0845 766 0163
Branches throughout the UK

National Survivor User Network
http://www.nsun.org.uk/
27–29 Vauxhall Grove, London, SW8 1SY, 0845 602 0779

Social Perspectives Network
http://www.spn.org.uk/

Survivors History Group
http://studymore.org.uk/mpu.htm

United Kingdom Advocacy Network
http://www.u-kan.co.uk/
c/o 8 Beulah View, Leeds, LS6 2LA

Index

LOVING CHRISTIAN

ONE FAMILY'S JOURNEY THROUGH SCHIZOPHRENIA

GEORGINA WAKEFIELD

ISBN 978 1 906254 30 8   2010
p. 195, £9.99 (£9.50 direct from www.pccs-books.co.uk)

A vivid, ultimately hopeful, personal account of a mother's struggle to understand and live positively with her son's stigmatising diagnosis of schizophrenia.

> *The story is a profound one that holds a mirror up to the structures of the society in which we live and just how easy it is to be disenfranchised from those structures if one moves away from the usual track of life's ups and downs. The story is also a critique for the mental health system itself. Incisive observations are offered as to what is the very best and worst of the system, telling examples of what needs to be put right in our own 'back yard'. Wakefield makes a plea for greater hope to be offered. I stand by her in making that plea and join with her in asking for recovery to be the theme for mental health care in this country.*

Professor Anthony Sheehan, former Director of Social Care for the Department of Health

PCCS BOOKS
w w w . p c c s - b o o k s . c o . u k

THIS IS SURVIVOR RESEARCH

ANGELA SWEENEY, PETER BERESFORD,
ALISON FAULKNER, MARY NETTLE & DIANA ROSE (EDS

ISBN 978 1 906254 14 8   2009
pp. 200, £20.00 (£18.00 direct from www.pccs-books.co.uk)

There has been a major development in health and social science
research: it is now being carried out by people who had previousl
only been seen as its subjects. At the forefront are people with
experience as mental health service users/survivors who have
taken a lead in pioneering a new approach to research which is
now commanding increasing attention and respect.

This is Survivor Research for the first time details this
important new approach to research. Written and edited by
leaders in the field it:

- explores the theory and practice of survivor research
- provides practical examples of survivor research, and
- offers guidance for people wishing to carry out such research
  themselves.

*This book is a major achievement. It helps us understand
exactly how far survivor-led research has taken us and how
much further there is to go. It also celebrates the enormous
achievements of the last 10 to 20 years. It is essential
reading for all those interested in mental health research,
whether it is survivor led, survivor informed or not. Surely
no one can question the substance or relevance of survivor-
led research after reading this book.*

Andrew McCulloch, Chief Executive of the Mental
Health Foundation

PCCS BOOKS
w w w . p c c s - b o o k s . c o . u k